*colds . . . cough . . . ulcers . . . impotence
. . . constipation . . . anemia . . . obesity . . .
arthritis . . . arteriosclerosis . . . warts . . . hair
loss . . . chronic fatigue . . .*

How do Oriental herbalists continue to diagnose and treat the major and minor afflictions familiar to us all, as they have for thousands of years? This book explains what is used and why in these and many other areas:

- Respiratory, digestive and circulatory conditions
- Urinary and genital problems
- Blood disorders
- Surgical and dermatological problems
- Ear, eye, nose and throat ailments
- Abnormal metabolism

The author, well known in this country and elsewhere, was trained in Japan and has been a herbologist for over 45 years. He indeed knows his subject well—and explains it thoroughly here for the Western reader.

ABOUT THE AUTHOR

Masaru Toguchi was born in Hawaii on July 17, 1915. At the age of thirteen, he started to learn herbology and acupuncture from his grandfather (Seiyu Kikuyama) in Okinawa, Japan. After his grandfather died in 1930, Toguchi returned to Hawaii. There, many people—knowing of his studies in herbs and acupuncture—sought him out for treatments. In 1952 he pursued extension courses with Dr. Ouchi of The Kawasaki Institute of Scientific Research in Tokyo. In 1955 he returned to the Institute, then specializing in radiological theory and electromagnetic therapeutics, and graduated in 1956. In 1958 he continued his studies at the Kato Acupuncture Hospital, Tokyo, where in 1959 he was awarded the Certificate of Keiketsugaku (neurology course of acupuncture) by Dr. Motayo Kato, president of the hospital. Toguchi holds a Certificate to Practice Massage, issued by the Board of Massage of Hawaii. Masaru Toguchi has used his methods successfully on numerous well-known entertainers.

ORIENTAL HERBAL WISDOM

MASARU TOGUCHI

CONSULTING EDITOR

Samuel Klein, Dr.Sc., Fellow,
Royal Society of Health

PYRAMID BOOKS   •   NEW YORK

ORIENTAL HERBAL WISDOM

A PYRAMID BOOK

First printing, July 1973

ISBN 0-515-02906-8

Printed in the United States of America

Pyramid Books are published by Pyramid Communications, Inc. Its trademarks, consisting of the word "Pyramid" and the portrayal of a pyramid, are registered in the United States Patent Office.

PYRAMID COMMUNICATIONS, INC.
919 Third Avenue
New York, New York 10022, U.S.A.

ORIENTAL
HERBAL
WISDOM

CONTENTS

FOREWORD

Although medical science has advanced by giant steps and the human life span has been lengthened, many people today still suffer from chronic disorders and incurable conditions. Discouraged by the frequently ineffectual means of modern medicine, many of these people are seeking out the advice of herbalists. Herbalism, which has lain dormant in Western countries since the advance of modern medical science, is beginning to emerge once again, and its true worth is becoming realized.

The Herbal Way, with a long history of proved results, was set aside in the awakening of modern technological civilization—not because herbal remedies were believed ineffective, but as possibly because pharmaceutical manufacturers found more profit in drugs that were easily synthesized in the laboratory than in herbals with a limited source of supply. Secondly, they could build a better sales pitch around mass-produced and easily dispensed "wonder drugs" than they could around herbal compositions that must be prepared on an individual basis. Thus healing values gradually became secondary to modern techniques of advertisement and profitmaking, as physicians tended routinely to choose pharmaceuticals and ignore the healthful properties of natural herbals.

The greatest advantage of herbals is that they are

organic—they have the same make-up as the food we eat every day. Therefore, the digestive mechanism of the human body, which is used to breaking down and absorbing natural things, can deal more smoothly with herbal materials than with man-made chemical structures, which are often more irritating. In other words, herbal medicines are not synthetic chemical compounds but natural foods that assist the body's healing abilities.

However, it must be emphasized that for the effective use of herb compositions close observation of the sick person's physical make-up and reactions is vital. The rules for administering herbals derive from experience in handling people over a long period of time. Herbal remedies are to be used by a person according to his physical structure: the dosages for two persons with the same condition probably will not be the same because of differences in their physical characteristics. Herbalists hardly ever use the same herbal in the same amount uniformly in the manner that present Western medicines are prescribed.

Countless numbers of herb compositions are known to the practicing herbalist. A herbal remedy can be suggested for almost every known condition.

The author does not intend to disseminate information about the application of herb compositions for the treatment of various diseases and bodily disorders. Rather, this book has been written for the purpose of explaining in brief the nature of herbalism in the Orient.

MASARU TOGUCHI, *Herbalist*

INTRODUCTION:
What is Herbalism?

Categorizing illnesses in the traditional Oriental Herbal way differs in many respects from modern medical science. Modern medical science stress the diagnosis of the illness and its cause while Chinese herbalism is based on the determination of the Sho (proof). The word *Sho* literally means "temperment" or "condition". Thus the Sho is the combination of symptoms: herbalism concentrates on the relief of symptoms and promotion of general health.

Oriental herbalism is the study of Sho. The proper herb is chosen according to the Sho, and Oriental herbalism has its own unique system of observing conditions and determining remedies. The Sho—the condition of the body—begins with the determination of a person as Yin, Yang, Kyo, or Jitsu (these terms describe general constitutional characteristics). The process for arriving at a conclusion of whether the person's Sho is Yin, Yang, Kyo, or Jitsu is unique to Oriental herbalism. After determination of the Sho, the herbal appropriate to the Sho can be used accurately.

The purposes of modern medical science are the prevention and treatment of illnesses. Concerning treatment, Oriental herbalism coincides naturally with the purposes of medical science. However, modern medical science in the West deals with sickness by placing the main emphasis on the study of the illness itself, thus spending too much time on testing, almost as though it has forgotten about treating the illness. Suppose there is a situation in which a person is made well by an herbal composition. A modern doctor might say that unless it is understood why the cure occurred, it has no value. Western doctors have long viewed the Oriental system of acupuncture with this attitude. Only recently have they begun to think acupuncture may have value —even if they do not comprehend *how* it works.

Oriental herbalism concerns itself little with the study of pathogens and other causes of illness. Modern medical science has strived to overcome this weakness, often with marked success; thus it has increased its influence and the Oriental herbalism approach—which centers its concern on the individual person rather than on causes—tends to be disregarded.

Today, many illnesses with unknown causes, such as neuralgia and rheumatism that produce pain when the weather gets cold and damp, headaches, stiff joints, and loss of steadiness of the legs and hips, baffle modern medical science and render it powerless with respect to treatment. In this area, the weakness of modern medical science has been gradually exposed in comparison with the strengths of Oriental herbalism in treating disorders with unknown causes.

Modern medical science and Oriental herbalism should be regarded as two sides of a shield. The shield offers full protection only if both sides are used to their best effect. By utilizing the special advantages of both modern medical science and Oriental herbalism—and by strengthening the weak points of both—sound medical science can be established for the sake of the health of mankind.

In modern medical science, it is impossible to prescribe the proper medicine if the name of the illness is undecided. Hence the key point in treatment is to diagnose correctly. One after the other, precision machines such as the X-ray machine, the electrocardiograph, and the electroencephalograph, have been developed for diagnostic purposes and made practical. Using the data supplied by these machines, the physician guesses at the name of the disease. This process of so-called scientific diagnosis involved an enormous effort to determine the name of the illness; the prescribed treatment —usually a mass-produced drug—is conveniently given according to the most advanced remedy for that illness available at that time. Of course, depending on experience, the physician uses some variation in selecting medicine and establishing dosages. However, we presume that almost identical dosages are prescribed to persons of varying physical structure and constitution. We believe that medicines are probably prescribed with little regard for the patient's basic constitution—i.e., whether the Sho is Kyo or Jitsu.

It is *not* necessary in Oriental herbalism to know the name of the illness in modern medical terms. Also, it is not necessary to maintain precision tools for the diagnosis of an illness or disorder. In other words, for the 20,000 years that have elapsed since the system of Oriental herbalism became established, herbalists have known how to employ an intuitive method of treatment (although it was still simplistic by the end of the Han Dynasty, A.D. 220). An old Oriental saying holds that "the reaction [symptoms] to an illness shows up on the body surface." It was thought that these external reactions were signs that could always be detected objectively through the five senses. Based on this conviction, the proper herbal was determined by relying only on the person's complaints in terms of certain reactions. Even today, the key point in determination is discerning the abnormal conditions that appear on the surface of the person's body.

In other words, the basic principle of treatment in modern medical science requires the accurate diagnosis of the name of the illness and considers it important to detect the various causes and to examine their functions. But in Oriental herbalism the determination of the name of the illness is not important; rather, the important preliminary to treatment is the reactions that need to be taken care of. Thus Oriental herbalism treats each person as an individual.

Some people nowadays feel it is unthinkable to dabble in outmoded remedies such as Oriental herbs. There are also those who feel that any doctor who studies something as unscientific as Oriental herbalism damages his stature as a medical practitioner.

The body of Oriental herbal knowledge has been passed down from ancient days. Its development was completed before the rise of modern medicine in Western Europe. Because the two approaches evolved separately, there are many aspects of Oriental herbalism that cannot be explained by the modern scientific method. Some parts of it even appear irrational and superstitious. But can we reject Oriental herbalism as unscientific? If the only medicine that is considered "scientific" is that which is measurable by the standards of modern medical science and if the rest are considered not worthy of research since they cannot be measured, then medical research will always remain at its current static level. Therefore, is it not a worthy mission for a medical doctor to study, with modern methods, the mysteries of herbalism unsolved by medical science and to find scientific explanations for their success? To study herbalism with the scientific method, in my opinion, will soon become an important objective of medical doctors all over the world.

The study of Oriental herbs is now gaining popularity in Germany and France, but not in an attempt to rebuild the old Oriental herbalism. The current study of Oriental herbs is aimed at creating a new medical science for tomorrow based upon the knowledge of the present and the past.

*　　　　　*　　　　　*

TRANSLATOR'S NOTE: Many of the passages, as they were translated, were expressed in a manner more readily understood by readers in English. For example, *Taiyobyo* and *Taiinbyo* should be written as *Daiyobyo* and *Daiinbyo*, but for phonetic consistency within this translation the former spelling is used. Also, words ending in "tsu" in combination with the ending "sho" normally are contracted to the combined form "-ssho," but again, for consistency, the words were not combined according to the rule for this translation—eg., "Jitsusho" instead of contracted form "Jissho."

Japanese words that have no equivalent in English are marked with an asterisk.

PART 1:

Oriental Herbal Determination

THERE ARE basic rules in Oriental herbalism for determining the Sho (the specific condition that is the objective of treatment) and the prescription (the method of treatment).

SHO

When the suffix *Sho* is attached to the name of a herbal, such as Kakkonto-sho (root of *Pueraria* brew), the term indicates that the condition calls for the herbal remedy called Kakkonto, showing that the potential for recovery is present if Kakkonto is given.

This type of determination is the foundation of Oriental herbalism. In modern medical science, by contrast, it is said that such and such symptoms exist for a certain ailment. But in Oriental herbalism, for example, Kakkonto-sho involves such and such reactions, and if these reactions exist, it is determined as Kakkonto-sho. Instead of determining it as such and such an illness, it is determined as such and such a Sho.

Yin and Yang

Much of Oriental philosophy favors a dualistic cosmic theory, of which the components are yin and yang. Yang is the male principle, which is active and light and symbolizes the heavens. Yin is the female principle, which is passive and dark and symbolizes the earth. If a person considers yin ($-$) and yang ($+$) as

17

negative and positive, then he will readily understand what they mean.

Yang-sho

A Yang-sho person has active and magnified reactions that tend to show up outwardly. For example, if he has a cold, his pulse becomes fast, his temperature goes up, his head aches, his body aches, his face flushes, he becomes thirsty, and he coughs violently.

Yin-sho

A Yin-sho person shows quiet and subdued reactions that tend to remain internal and are slow to appear. For example, if an old person or a frail child catches a cold, he just lies there without much energy and looks pale. He shows no fever, his pulse is weak and slow, and he does not even cough. At first his condition does not seem serious. However, a Yin-sho person has more difficulty in responding to a herbal than a Yang-sho person does. His recovery is slow. A Yang-sho person can use strong, aggressive herbals such as sweat producers and fever reducers, but a Yin-sho person must use heat-giving herbals that allow him to retain warmth.

Kyo and Jitsu

Kyo describes a person who is constitutionally frail. *Jitsu* describes a person who is strong, energetic, and full of vitality.

Kyokyo-sho

If a person feels chilly or cold, has a weak pulse, has a headache and stiff shoulders, and perspires naturally, then he is Kyokyo-sho. In this case the herbalist suggests the use of Keishito (cinnamon bark brew).

Rikyo-sho

This person has a soft belly with no muscles, lacks vigor, has no appetite, and is bothered by diarrhea. He feels either heavy in the stomach or sick in the stomach and complains of nausea. His pulse is weak. If such reactions exist, the condition is Rikyo-sho. For such a person, the herbalist suggests that he should take Shinbuto, Ninjinto (ginseng brew), or Shigyakuto for warmth and strength.

Hyojitsu-sho

This person feels chilly or cold, has a headache, and does not perspire naturally even if he has a fever. His pulse is fast. With such reactions, he is said to have Hyojitsu-sho. For such Sho, the herbalist will use Maoto (Ephedra brew) or Kakkonto to stimulate perspiration.

Rijitsu-sho

This person feels heavy in the belly and constipated, gets a yellow coating on his tongue, and complains of thirst. He has a subdued but strong pulse. With such reactions, he is said to be Rijitsu-sho. For such Sho, the herbalist suggests Daisaikoto (Large *Bupleurum* brew) or Daijokito to flush out and clean the stomach.

Hyokyorijitsu-sho

This person is constipated and feels full in the belly. If his pulse is subdued but strong, his condition is Rijitsu-sho. But if, in addition, chills accompany the above reactions, the condition is Hyokyorijitsu-sho. For such Sho the herbalist will use Keishito first to relieve Hyokyo and then Daisaikoto to relieve Rijitsu.

This person has chills and a fever; his body aches. He may have diarrhea more than ten times a day. These reactions occur because his Kyo-sho is both Hyo and Ri. For this condition the herbalist will give first Shigyakuto to relieve Rikyo-sho, then Keishito to relieve Kyokyo-sho.

Kitai-sho

Kitai-sho is determination by means of the movements of the body fluids. Ki has no form but only movement: it is the force that moves blood and water within the body. If Ki is languid, the blood and water also become sluggish. When such reactions are present, therefore, herbal compositions are administered to offset the poisons that remain in the blood and water because the fluids are not moved quickly enough through the lungs and kidneys.

Herbals to regulate the Ki movement are called Kitai. When a person becomes ill, Ki tends to rise. When Ki rises, his feet become cold, and his face flushes with fever; he has headaches, dizzy spells, and fast palpitations. In such a case, the herbalist would use Keishito.

Furthermore, the person affected with such an illness feels depressed. Therefore, the herbalist will give Hangekobokuto (*Pinella-Magnolia* brew) to disperse the depression. Depression affects water and blood circulation. Therefore, in the composition the herbalist will include herbals that are effective for alleviating depression in addition to using herbals for Ki. Even with the use of Daijokito, a herbal useful for regulating mood, Koboku (*Magnolia*) is mixed in to improve Ki.

Oketsu-sho

The concept of Oketsu is unique to Oriental herbalism and is commonly called "old blood." But *Oketsu* actually means *stagnation of the blood*.

Oketsu cannot adequately be described in Western terminology. However, it can be determined that Oketsu exists when the following reactions are present: The mouth is dry; the person wants to wet his mouth, but he does not feel like drinking. His stomach is not full, but it feels like it is full. He feels feverish either all over his body or locally. His skin or mucous membrane has purple spots. Blue veins appear on his skin, or his skin resembles that of a shark. Around the edges of his tongue, a dark purple color appears, and the lips become blue. His stool appears black. He bleeds easily. When the Sho is confirmed as Oketsu, the herbalist will select one remedy from among Tokeishokito*, Keiryogan*, Taiobotanhito*, and Teitogan*.

Tanin-sho

Phlegm in Oriental herbalism is different from *sputum* in modern medical science. *Phlegm* means *water* and represents body fluid. Sputum, of course, is included in such a definition. Phlegm is also called *Tanin*, and both terms represent water poison.

Ancient people said, "Kaitan (mysterious phlegm) must be treated as Tan (phlegm)." This saying means that abnormalities that are difficult to determine should be treated as abnormalities of water.

The human body is about 70 percent water. When

* Japanese words that have no equivalent in English are marked with an asterisk throughout—translation

21

water metabolism is interrupted and the smooth flow of circulatory distribution is lost, various reactions develop. Also, when external conditions cause interruption of water metabolism, rheumatism may develop. Abnormalities caused by changes in water flow often accompany blood conditions and simultaneous changes in general health. The most common reactions indicative of Tanin-sho include sloshing noises below the heart, growling noises in the stomach, diarrhea, nausea, constipation, decreased urination, excessive urination, swelling, palpitations, dizziness, tinnitus aurium, headaches, sputum, excessive secretion of saliva, pains in the joints, asthma, coughing, dryness of the mouth, excessive perspiration, and body sweating.

Herbals used most frequently to control water metabolism are Bukuryoin (*Pachyma*), Tokisha (*Alisma*), Choreito (*Chuling**), Mokutsu (*Akebia*), Maoto (*Ephedra*), and Saishin (*Asarum*).

Boshin

Using the method of determination called Boshin, even without medical training, one can fairly easily make a rough determination as to the yin, yang, kyo, and jitsu of a person. Boshin may be defined as a method of determination by external observation of the person, taking into account his skeletal, muscular, and skin characteristics.

If a person has a solid bone structure and good nutritional condition, his muscles are not flabby, and he is heavy built, he is Jitsu-sho in most cases. For such Jitsu-sho, there are more opportunities to use Daisai Koto (Large *Bupleurum*), Bofutsukensan*, and Daijokito.

If, however, the person is fat and flabby—that is, if he is bloated with water and his skin color is pale, his bone structure delicate, and his skin texture smooth, then he is Kyo-sho in most cases. Herbals such as Boio-gito (*Astragalus* brew), which includes Oki (*Astragalus*), or a combination of Kyu (*Atractylodes* rhizome) and Bukuryo (*Pachyma*) are frequently used by the herbalist; if determination of this person is mistaken as Jitsu-sho and he is given a laxative mixed with Daio (*Rheum*), he will only become exhausted.

Many people who are considered Kyo-sho are skinny and have a bad complexion. However, there are exceptions to this rule; and if the Sho is determined by external appearances alone, the determination will go wrong. It is necessary to determine the Sho based on over-all observations, not just external reactions. If the patient is thin but his flesh is tight and his complexion is dark, herbals such as Shinbutsuto*, Hachimiganryo, and Jiinkokato*, which are mixed with Jio (*Rehmannia*), are often used by the herbalist. If the person's face looks red and blood easily rushes to his head, herbals such as Sanoshashinto and Orengedokuto (*Coptis* laxative brew), which are mixed with Oren (*Coptis*) and Hoshi (*Gardenia*), are used by the herbalist. Paleness with a tinge of reddish color, as seen on the face of a tubercular person, was known to ancient people as *Kyokajoen,* and a herbal that included Bakumonto (*Ophiopogon*) and Gomishi (*Schizandra*) was used for this Sho.

If, as a result of stagnation of the blood, the body becomes reddish-pink and capillary vessels become visible like a net, Haikakujokito*, which clears stagnated blood, is used by the herbalist.

An old person, a person recovering from a serious illness, a diabetic person, or a person with atrophied kidneys can have dry skin, just like a dead leaf. Since this phenomenon is caused by loss of nutrition in body fluids, the herbalist provides herbals such as Ninjinto (ginseng), Chiojio (*Anemarrhena-Rehmannia*), Shak-

23

uyaku (*Paeonia*), and Toki Tokishakuyaku sanyro (*Liguesticum*), which are effective in supplying nutrition.

Zetsu-sho

Zetsu-sho is determination by means of observing the condition of the tongue. Healthy persons do not have a coating on their tongue. Taiyobyo (big yang illness) with Hyo-sho shows no coating on the tongue. Also, Inbyo (yin illness) shows moisture on the tongue without a coating. Various other conditions without fever often show no coating on the tongue.

Hakutai (White Coating)

When a white coating appears on the tongue that had not been observed previously and when the saliva becomes sticky, accompanied by thirstiness, it indicates that Taiyobyo has changed into Shoyobyo (little yang illness). The reactions indicate the appropriate treatment is Shosaikoto. When a white coating appears on the tongue, laxatives should not be used. Use Shosaikoto (Little *Bupleurum* brew), Jiokoto*, Hangeshashinto, Orento (*Coptis* brew), or Shokankyoto*.

Otai (Yellow Coating)

When Hakutai changes into Otai, purging the bowels may be effective in some cases but may be bad in other cases. When Hakutai gradually becomes yellow from the center of the tongue out—but before Otai becomes thick—do not purge too hastily. As time passes, Otai changes into a brownish color and the appropriate treatment is a laxative. However, in this case, the pulse should be taken (Myaku-sho, see below) and abdomen examined (Fuku-sho, see below) before purging the bowels. In general, a herbalist will use Daisaikoto (Large *Bupleurum* brew).

Kokutai (Black Coating)

When a black coating appears on the tongue, the appropriate herbal may be a laxative. Or the condition may be Kyo-sho and require warm heat applications (rinsing of mouth with warm fluid). If the tongue is brownish-black due to fever, pinch the tongue with the fingers to see if it is hard. If it is hard, purge the bowels since it is a jitsu fever; in this case, the herbalist will use Jiokito*. If the tongue is black and dry but it is soft to the touch, a laxative should not be taken; the herbalist will use Shigyakuto* or Ninjinto (ginseng brew).

When the person has a high fever, he cannot see clearly, his tongue is brownish-black, he cannot talk, his hearing is poor, and he shows pain when his stomach is pressed in, the condition is Jitsu-sho and calls for a laxative.

On the other hand, if the tongue is soft and the person is able to stick it out even though he appears to be in a daze, is unable to talk, and can't feel food in his mouth, Kyo-sho is indicated and he should not use a laxative.

If the coating is black, thick, and dry, his lips are cracked, and even his gums are black and dry, and if he feels pain when pressed in the area below the heart, Jitsu-sho is indicated and he may be purged with a laxative. If, however, no coating is seen on the tongue but the tongue is black all over, laxatives are not applicable.

If the tongue has lost the papillae from its surface and is plainly red and dry, the Sho calls for nutritive herbals such as Jio (*Rehmannia*), Bakumonto (*Ophiopogon*), Chimo (*Anemarrhena*), and Ninjinto (gins-

25

eng). An old man, or a woman after childbirth, often has this type of Jitsu-sho.

If the tongue is dark purple or blue or if there are blotches around the edges of the tongue, it is a type of Jitsu-sho indicating Oketsu (stagnation of blood).

MONSHIN

Monshin, or determination by questioning, is employed to find out how the patient feels. The herbalist may begin by asking the person how he feels with regard to chill, cold, fever. Then the herbalist may also question the person about aches, pains, dizziness, stiffness, and other reactions the herbalist cannot discover by his own objective examination.

Chill and Cold

Chill is an internal feeling, and cold is an external feeling. Chill means that the person feels chilly even after he warms himself. Cold means a person feels an unpleasant lack of warmth only when the air temperature is too low or when he is out in the wind. Both chill and cold are reactions characteristic of Hyo-sho. Therefore, it is important to ask the person about these reactions without fail in order to determine whether the condition of Hyo-sho is present. Note that the person with chills or who is cold is not necessarily Hyo-sho.

The condition in which chill and fever exist simultaneously, is a sign of Hyo-sho. If the chill disappears and the fever goes up, (alternating cold and fever) the reaction is a type of fever characteristic of Shoyobyo (little yang illness).

For chill and fever the herbalist will use a herbal for Hyo-sho, such as Keishito, Maoto, or Kakkonto, while alternating cold and fever is a type of fever that requires Shikozai (*Bupleurum* herb).

26

Kantaiyobyo (perspiration accompanying big yang illness) is Hyo-sho. Natural sweating occurs without the use of sweat herbs and is indicative of Hyokyo. Keishito (cinnamon bark brew) should be used. However, even if the fever is Hyokyo, there may be a period in which the person does not sweat. In this case the differentiation must be made by taking the pulse. In the case of Hyokyo, the pulse is weak. In the case of Hyojitsu, no natural sweating occurs and the pulse is strong.

Basically, Inbyo (yin illness) is not accompanied by sweating. If sweat pours out, it is called Dakken (profuse sweating) and is indicative of a serious illness.

Fever

In Oriental herbalism, fever (Netsu) does not always imply a rise in body temperature. A feverish feeling without measurable rise in body temperature is also considered to be a fever; this feverish feeling on the body surface may feel feverish to the touch of others.

A fever alone may indicate *either* Hyo-sho or Ri-sho; if a chill occurs simultaneously, the condition is Hyo-sho.

In general, alternating cold and fever means cold and fever occur alternately; when the chill stops, the fever increases, and when the fever stops, the chill takes over. This type of fever is characteristic of Shoyobyo (little yang illness).

Chonetsu (tide fever) is diagnosed when the fever spreads all over the body and is not accompanied by a chill; at the same time the person perspires from the top of his head to the tips of his fingers and toes. If his feet get cold or if perspiration develops on his head only, the reaction cannot be designated as Chonetsu. Chonetsu is a type of fever related to Yomeibyo (yan

27

ming* illness), and a laxative will be suggested by the herbalist.

Shinnetsu (body fever) is similar to Chonetsu in that the whole body becomes feverish; however, there is no perspiring of the whole body. Shinnetsu is also a type of fever related to Yomeibyo.

In the case of Shusokuhannetsu (fever of hands and feet), the hands and feet feel hot and the person prefers to leave them uncovered and likes to touch cool objects. In this case, Jiozai (*Rehmannia* herbal) is usually used by the herbalist; no laxatives should be taken.

Stool

Persons who are constipated and produce hard stools are in most cases Jitsu-sho. Those who have diarrhea or soft bowels are Kyo-sho although there are exceptions to this rule. Some persons who are Kyo-sho do get constipated. Even if a person feels congestion in his stomach and is constipated, his pulse may be weak with no strength in his abdomen. In this case, the bowel movement can be restored through heat-giving and nutritive herbs.

If a person is constipated due to a fever and has a weak pulse, he is Kyo-sho. If Daio (*Rheum*) or Shisho (*sodium sulfate*) laxatives are used, he loses vigor. If Shigyakuto or Shinbuto is given for providing warmth, the person will regain strength in his stomach and have natural bowel movements.

If a person has diarrhea but the area below the heart remains hard and is painful, the condition is Jitsu-sho and in many cases Daisaikoto (Large *Bupleurum* brew) is used. If the diarrhea is severe and repetitious, the condition is Jitsu-sho, and it is often necessary for the herbalist to use preparations that include Daio (*Rheum*) and Shakuyaku (*Paeonia*).

When the stool is black, the cause may be Oketsu

28

(stagnated blood). If the stool has a bad odor and is viscous, the condition is generally Jitsu-sho. However, if the stool is hard and dry like that of a rabbit, it is not suited to laxate; rather, the Sho calls for nutritive herbs such as Ninjin (ginseng) or Jio (*Rehmannia*). If the stool is bluish or pale without viscosity—i.e., of the diarrhea type—without the ordinary odor, the condition is Kyo-sho and the herbalist will use Kankyo (dried rhizome of *Zingiber*).

Urination

Shobenfuri means a small amount of urination. Shobenjiri means excessive urination. Shobennan means urination is difficult.

Shobenfuri has distinctions as Kyo and Jitsu—that is, the condition may be mild or severe. In many conditions, as a result of perspiration, diarrhea, bleeding, vomiting, etc., body fluids are reduced and Shobenfuri can develop. In such a case, nothing in particular need be done to increase urination.

As an early sign of conditions called Osoku or Fushu, Shobenfuri may occur. In such cases, Kokatsu (dryness in the mouth) develops. The herbal Inchinkoto (*Artemisia* brew) or Goreisan is given by the herbalist. If, on the other hand, there is no swelling but body fluids are poorly distributed, Shobenfuri can develop. In such a case, the herbalist will use a herbal mixture of Bukuryo (*Pachyma*), Jitsu (*Atractylodes* rhizome), Takusha (*Alisma*), and Chorei (*Chuling*).

Persons who have Shobenjiri are generally Yin-sho and Kyo-sho. The Sho mostly calls for Hachimiganryo, Shokenchuto, Ryokyojutukanto*, and Kansokankyoto (*Laquititia*-dried rhizome of *Zingiber* brew). Shobenfuri can also occur as a result of Oketsu (blood stagnation).

Kokatsu (Thirst)

Kokatsu is an abnormal thirst. When the thirst is severe, it is called Hankatsuinin. Persons who complain of Kokatsu may be divided into those who have dry lips as well as dry tongues and those who have moist tongues. Also, there are those who prefer hot water and others who prefer cold water. Furthermore, there are those who have dry mouths and little saliva and who want to wet their mouths but do not wish to drink water; this reaction is called Kokan and is distinguished from Kokatsu.

Hankatsuinin may be either Yang-sho or Yin-sho. To distinguish between these two, the herbalist looks for Myaku-sho (pulse) or other references before making a determination.

When a person prefers hot water, he is said to be Yin-sho, and when he prefers cold water, he is said to be Yang-sho. But the terms in this case are merely descriptive and that is all. We should not separate the Sho as yang or yin. For even a Yin-sho at its most extreme would conversely cause a person to wish to drink cold water, as if the condition had changed to Yang-sho. The Yang-sho, too, at its extreme may cause a preference for hot water.

For Yang-sho, a herbal such as Byakkoto* containing Sekko (gypsum) is used; while for Yin-sho, herbals such as Shinbuto and Bukuryoshigyakuto* are used by the herbalist. When Kokatsu is not severe, nutritional herbals such as Shorokon* Ninjin (ginseng), Chimo (*Anemarrhena*), and Jio (*Rehmannia*) are used.

Kokatsu has no Jitsu-sho but only Kyo-sho. However, Kokan may be brought on as a result of Oketsu (blood stagnation). It is imperative that the Sho be clearly understood by comparing it with other Sho.

With the exception of Oketsu, heat-giving and nutritional herbals are applied.

For example, a seriously ill person or an old person may wake up after a nap with such a thirst that he can hardly move his tongue unless he drinks water. Such a condition indicates a Sho calling for Ninjin (ginseng), Bukuryoin (*Pachyma*), and Jio (*Rehmannia*).

Kokan caused by taking chemical drugs must be carefully distinguished so that the proper antidote may be administered.

Coughs

When a person has a cough, the herbalist must find out if he also wheezes, if it is a dry cough or a wet cough, if the phlegm is easy or difficult to cough out, and if the quantity of phlegm is large or small. It is also necessary to find out if he has to cough until his face becomes red, if he feels dry deep inside of his throat, if he coughs more often when he uses a heater, and if he coughs badly at night or more frequently in the morning.

For wheezing coughs, a herbal mixed with Maoto (*Ephedra*) is often used by the herbalist. A dry cough has no phlegm. At the early stages of a dry cough Maoto (*Ephedra*) is again used; however, if a dry cough continues for a while, the Jio (*Rehmannia*), Bakumonto (*Ophipogon* brew), and Shakanzoto are used. However, if the phlegm is easy to cough out but its quantity is large and the coughing becomes more serious, the amount of phlegm will increase if nutritive herbals, such as those mentioned above are used. When the inside of the throat becomes dry or when the coughing increases when a heater is used, the condition is suited to nutritive herbals.

If the coughing is accompanied by Hyo-sho, a herbalist can stop the coughing by using herbals for Hyo-sho. However, if the coughing continues after Hyo-sho has left, then the herbals must be given according to the Sho.

Bleeding

Although a person with fever and congestion may bleed, if his hands and feet remain warm, his complexion good, and his pulse strong, the herbalist can give Sanoshashinto or Orengedokuto, which contain Oren (*Coptis*).

On the other hand, if the person's hands and feet become cold, his complexion bad, and his pulse weak with a cold constitution or Oketsu (blood stagnation), the herbalist would use Kyukikyogaito, whose main ingredient is Jio (*Rehmannia*). However, there are times when these two conditions are mixed. In this case, the herbalist would use Onkoin*, which is a combination of Shinbutsuto* and Orengedokuto.

When bleeding is heavy and an anemic condition prevails, the herbalist will use Kokusanto* and Shikunshito* with the ingredient Ninjin (ginseng).

Apart from the above cases, bleeding may occur as a result of Oketsu. By referring to other signs, make sure which type of bleeding it is. If bleeding is caused by Oketsu, the herbalist will use Tokeijokito* and Sesshoin*.

Headaches

Different kinds of headaches are characteristic of yang, kyo, and jitsu. If a person has a headache, fever, and chill with a strong pulse, he has a headache characteristic of Taiyobyo (big yang illness), which indicates a Sho requiring Maoto (*Ephedra* brew). This is called a Hyo-sho headache. Conversely, although a person may have a headache, it may be a Sho requiring Maosaishinbushito (*Ephedra-Asarum* brew).

If the headache is so severe that a person vomits, his hands and feet turn cold, he becomes irritable, and his pulse becomes slow and subdued, this headache is also part of Inbyo-sho.

If a person with gastric atony or gastroptosis has a sloshing-water noise in the area below his heart, his feet turn cold, his shoulders and neck are stiff, he feels dizzy and he has a headache, the herbalist would use Hangebyakujutsutenmato.

Those who have Kyokyokuman (distressing fullness in the hypochondrium region) or Shingehiko (hardness in the region below the heart) often complain of reactions of heavy-headedness and headaches. In Oriental herbalism this is called Zucho (heavy-headedness). In this case, if Kyokyokuman exists, the herbalist chooses from among Shosaikoto (Little *Bupleurum* brew), and Saikokaryukotsuboreito (*Bupleurum–Os stegodontis–Ostrea* testa brew); if Shingehiko exists, he chooses between Hangeshinto and Sanoshashinto.

Dizziness

A patient with dizziness (Mokugen) usually has stiff shoulders at the same time. These stiff shoulders are generally caused by Kyokyokuman, Shingemanshin (fullness in the region below the heart), or Shingehiko. If a person complains of Kyokyokuman, the herbalist uses Shinkozai*; if he has Shingehiko and constipation, the herbalist will use Sanoshashinto. If there is also a sloshing noise in the stomach, he will use Reikeijutsukanto, Hangebyakujutsutenmato, Shinbuto, or Tokishakuyakusanryo (*Ligusticum-Paeonia* powder).

SESSHIN

Sesshin means that the herbalist uses his hands directly in contact with the patient's body in order to make a determination. Among these types of contact, the important ones are Myakushin and Fukushin.

Myakushin

Myakushin is determination by means of evaluating the pulse (Myaku). The pulse is taken by the herbalist at the same point that is used in modern medical science—that is, the pulsation of the radial artery in the wrist measured on the inside of the styloid process of the radius. Place the forefinger, the middle finger, and the third finger on this region and take the pulse. The pulse felt by the forefinger is called Sunko; that felt by the middle finger, Kanjo; and that felt by the third finger, Tenchyu. While taking the pulse the three fingers should touch each other lightly. If the person has a long forearm, spread the fingers a little; if he has a short arm, close the fingers a little.

The Purpose of Myakushin

The purpose of Myakushin is to learn the location of the illness; to know the yin, yang, kyo, and jitsu; to know how cold or feverish the person is; to identify the Sho; to know the past and present condition of the illness; and to know the general physiological condition of the person.

Some Types of Pulses

1. Fu: a pulse that seems to float on the surface (indicates location of illness is close to the surface).
2. Chin: a pulse detected by pressing down hard (indicates location of illness is internal).
3. Su: a fast pulse (indicates a fever within).
4. Chi: a slow pulse (indicates yin and kyo).
5. Gen: a strong pulse like the snapping of a bowstring (the pulse of Shoyobyo—little yang illness).

6. Kin: a delicate but strong pulse (indicates jitsu, pain, or cold).
7. Katsu: a smooth pulse (indicates a fever or jitsu).
8. Shoku or Ju: a hesitant pulse (indicates kyo).
9. Bi: a barely detectable pulse (indicates a loss of vitality).
10. Ko or Dai: a thick pulse (indicates a fever).
11. Ko: a hollow, thin weak pulse like the leaves of an onion (indicates an atrophied condition after a loss of blood).
12. Fun: a deep, internal pulse (indicates jitsu).
13. Jyaku or Nan: a weak pulse (indicates kyo).
14. Sai or Sho: a thin pulse (indicates yin or kyo).
15. Soku: a fast but irregular pulse (indicates yang).
16. Kettai: a slow and halting pulse (indicates yang or kyo, also irregular pulses).
17. Cho: a long pulse (indicates jitsu).
18. Tan: a short pulse (indicates kyo).
19. Kan: a pulse that is neither fast nor slow and indicates a calm, medium heartbeat; when a Kan pulse is detected in an illness, the illness is not serious and recovery is on its way.

Fukushin

Fukushin is the method of determination by means of probing the abdomen. The Fuku-sho is the condition of the abdomen. The herbalist will make the person lie down on his back, stretch his legs out straight and either place his hands at his sides or clasp his hands over his chest. The person should be relaxed so that he does not tighten up his stomach muscles before examination.

If the person tightens up his stomach muscles the determination will be mistakenly made as Kyokyokuman (distressing fullness in the hypochondrium region) or Rikyo of Fukuchokkin (contraction of tight-stretching straight muscles of the abdomen-recti abdomini), and

35

also will often make it impossible to hear the sloshing-water noises below the heart. It is therefore necessary to carry out Fukushin with the person's legs stretched out and then to repeat Fukushin with his legs bent at the knees so that the straight muscles of the abdomen are relaxed.

The Purpose of Fukushin

The purpose of Fukushin in Oriental herbalism is to determine kyo and jitsu. However, if the determination of kyo and jitsu is done through Fukushin alone, the possibility exists for a faulty determination. It is therefore necessary to refer to Myakushin and other reactions and to make overall observations.

Fuku-sho

If a person has an overall softness of the stomach and it has no strength and no resilience, if he has a weak and subdued pulse, and if his hands and feet are cold, the condition is Rikyo-sho; such Sho requires Shin-buto, Ninjinto (ginseng brew), and Shkunshito. In this case, even if there is a sloshing noise, it is still Rikyo-sho and requires the same herbals.

When the stomach is soft and weak, the intestines have peristaltic irregularity, and through the abdominal wall the peristaltic motion of the intestines can be felt. In this case, the condition is also Kyo-sho and the Sho requires Daikenchuto, Shokenchuto, Shinbuto, and Sen-pukukadai-chosekito* (a brew of *Inula* root and soluble iron salts).

When the stomach is soft but feels strong, the condition is Jitsu-sho. If a person is constipated and the pulse is subdued but strong, the Sho is suited to a laxative even though the stomach is soft and weak; Sano-shashinto is the herbal of choice.

Fukuman can be either Kyo-sho or Jitsu-sho. Jitsu-sho is more often the case in a person with Fukuman and constipation. If a person has Fukuman and his stomach has no strength and sags, the condition is Kyo-sho.

When a person purges his bowels and yet feels that his stomach is bloated, the condition is Kyo-sho. It is also Kyo-sho if, after a loss of body fluids, the person develops Fukuman. A person who has Fukuman and yet has basic strength in the area of his abdomen, and who may be constipated and yet have a strong pulse is Jitsu-sho. When a person has Fukuman but the surface of the stomach is hard with no basic strength in the area of the abdomen and if his pulse is weak, then his condition is Kyo-sho.

For persons with Jitsu-sho, the herbalist will use Daisaikoto (Large *Bupleurum* brew), Daijokito, and Inchinkoto (*Artemisia* brew), which contains Daio (*Rheum*) to purge the bowels. For those with Kyo-sho, the herbalist will use Keishikashakuyakuto (cinnamon bark–*Paeonia* brew), Shokenchuto, and Shigyakuto for warmth.

A person with gastroptosis or gastric atony often has the symptom of sloshing-water noises in the region below the heart. Such a person is, in most cases, Hyo-sho. Herbals such as Buryoin (*Pachyma-Alisma* brew) and Hangekobokuto (*Pinella-Magnolia* brew), which are mixtures of Bukuryo (Pachyma), Jutsu (rhizome of *Atractylodes*), Takusha (*Alisma*), Shoki (*Zingiber*), and Hange (*Pinella*), are used by the herbalist.

Shingehiko

The reaction called Shingehiko can be defined as a feeling of pressure resulting from a fullness in the region below the heart. *Hi* (from Shingehiko) means pressure. Frequently used herbals for Shingehiko are Hangeshashinto, Kanzoshashinto*, and Sanoshashinto.

Shingehi

Shingehi is a reaction commonly described as a feeling of something pushing out from the pit of the stomach. There is no sign of resistance or oppressive pain in this region detectable by others. A person with Shingehi often hears a sloshing-water noise. In most cases, Shingehi appears as Kyo-sho. Frequently, Shikunshito* and Ninjinto (ginseng brew) are used by the herbalist.

Kyokyokuman

As discussed previously, Kyokyokuman is a congested feeling at the hypochondrium; the feeling is distressing. The pressure and pain when this area is pressed can be sensed clearly by others. Kyokyokuman appears on both sides, but it may also appear only on one side (left or right). In most cases, Kyokyokuman is suited to such herbals such as Shinkozai*, (which contains *Bupleurum*). When the liver or the spleen is enlarged, it may be regarded as Kyokyokuman, but Shinkozai* is useless for cancer of the liver.

Kyogehiko

Kyogehiko is a congested hardening below the hypochondrium. In many cases, it occurs simultaneously with Kyokyokuman. The administration of Shinkozai* is appropriate.

Rikyu

Rikyu means a feeling of contraction underneath the abdominal skin. Contractions of Fukuchokkin (tight-stretching straight muscles of the abdomen) are included in this definition, as is the feeling of the stomach being full and stretched without the contraction of Fukuchokkin. Rikyu occurs among Kyo-sho patients. Since this is Fuku-sho, no laxative should be used even if a person is constipated. For Rikyu, Shokenhanto* and Daikenhanto* are used.

Shofukukokyu

Shofuku means lower abdomen. Shofukukokyu means the lower abdomen is in a contracted condition. In this case, Fukuchokkin is contracted from the navel on down to the pubic bone. This is frequently observed when Kyo of Kasho* develops. In other words, this is Fuku-sho, due to kidney trouble. This Sho is often found in Hachimigan-sho.

Shofukukyuketsu

Shofukukyuketsu is the Fuku-sho for Togakujokito; that is, it is Fuku-sho resulting from Oketsu (blood stagnation). This Fuku-sho seldom appears on the right side. When light pressure is applied to the iliac cavity on the left side, a ropy object the size of a pencil or finger, which gives increasing pain, is probed for. In order to examine this Fuku-sho, it is necessary to have the person stretch his legs out straight before examination. As the tips of the fingers touch the abdominal wall lightly, they are moved quickly as if rubbing from the navel diagonally toward the node of the left ilium. In this case, if Shofukukyuketsu exists, the person will suddenly bend his knees and complain of severe pain. This Fuku-sho exists more among women than men.

Shofukuman means the expansion of the lower abdomen. Shofukukoman means that after the lower abdomen expands, pressure exists. This Fuku-sho often appears as Oketsu-sho (stagnated blood) but it also appears as Tanin-sho (body fluids). Furthermore, the abdomen is hard and Shobenfuri (too little urination) occurs; this is called bloodlessness. When Shobenjiri (excessive urination) accompanies Shofukukoman, the condition is called Ketsu-sho (blood). In the case of Oketsu, a herbalist will use Keishibukuryogan (cinnamon bark–*Pachyma* pills), Daiobotanipito (*Rheum-Moutan* bark brew), and Teitogan*. In the case of Tanin-sho he will use Choreito (*Chuling* brew).

Shinki, Shinkaki, and Saikaki

Shinki means palpitation of the heart. When we say that the motion of Kyori (rapid heartbeat) accelerates, it means palpitation of the heart. When we speak of the motion that is taking place among Shinkaki*, Saikaki*, moisture, and kidneys, we mean that we can observe externally the abdominal pulsation of the main artery and also that we are able to feel it easily with our hands.

When the palpitation accelerates in these regions, they are all Kyo-sho, and therefore perspiration, purging, and vomiting must be avoided. Herbals for palpitations include ingredients such as Jio (*Rehmannia*), Bukuryo (*Pachyma*), Ryukotsuborei (*Os stegodontis* and Ostrea testa), Keishi (cinnamon bark), and Kanso (*Laquiritia*). For example, there are Saikanto, Keishikaryukotsuboreito, Ryokyojutsukanto, Ryokeikansoto, Hangekobokuto, and Goreisan.

THREE YINS–THREE YANGS

General unspecified conditions are classified as yin, yang, kyo, and jitsu in order to be treated. However, it is more convenient to use the Three Yins–Three Yangs classification for the treatment of Shokan, that is, an acute fever. According to the Shokan theory, the Three Yins–Three Yangs classification is used for an illness depending on how far it has progressed.

Taiyobyo

At the early stages of a fever, there are many conditions that start with the reactions of Taiyobyo (big yang illness). Therefore, from the Shokan theory, the following can generally be stated: Taiyobyo consists of Fumyaku ("floating on the surface" pulse), headaches, severe pain, and chill.

These four reactions characterize Taiyobyo. So, if all four of these reactions are present, regardless of the name of the condition, it is called Taiyobyo. On the other hand, if the condition is called Taiyobyo, is it always necessary to have all four reactions present? We find that this is not always so. Here are a couple of examples. The most important one among the four reactions of Taiyobyo is Fumyaku. However, just because the pulse is Fu (floating) does not necessarily mean the condition is Taiyobyo. The reason is that although it rarely occurs, Shoyobyo (little yang illness), Yomeibyo (yang ming illness), Taiinbyo (big yin illness), and Shoinbyo (little yin illness) can also have Fumyaku. Therefore, in addition to this Fumyaku, there must be another related reaction that characterizes Taiyobyo. Otherwise we cannot define it as Taiyobyo.

Although headaches are also characteristic of the reactions of Taiyobyo, with headaches alone, the condition cannot be called Taiyobyo. A similar argument can also be used for severe pain and chill.

Thus it becomes apparent that Taiyobyo is determined depending on which reactions are combined with the others.

If the pulse is Fu and is accompanied by a fever and chill, the condition is Taiyobyo. If the pulse is Fu together with a fever, cold, and headache, the condition is Taiyobyo. If the pulse is Fu accompanied by a fever, chill, and body pains, the condition is Taiyobyo. If the pulse is Fu together with a fever, headache, chill, and pain in the joints, the condition is Taiyobyo.

Reactions of Taiyobyo appear on the surface of the body, and therefore they coincide with the reactions of Hyo-sho.

For the treatment of Taiyobyo, Keishito (cinnamon bark brew), Maoto (*Ephedra* brew), and Kakkonto (*Pueraria* root brew) are used by the herbalist.

Shoyobyo

When a condition starts out as Taiyobyo but after three or four days changes to Shoyobyo (little yang illness), the following reactions occur: a bitterness inside the mouth, a dryness in the throat, and dizziness in the eyes. These characteristics of Shoyobyo are all subjective reactions, and only by Monshin (determination by questioning) can they be detected. The reaction of bitterness in the mouth is caused by the fever, and the mouth tends to become sticky at the same time.

There is no reaction of bitterness in the mouth for Taiyobyo and the three yin conditions. However, Yomeibyo (yang ming* conditions) may cause bitterness in mouth. Hence, with such a reaction alone, it is difficult to differentiate between Yomeibyo and Shoyobyo (little yang illness). In order to distinguish between these conditions, we need to consider the

Fuku-sho (condition of the abdomen) and other reactions. Inkan means a feeling of dryness in the throat, but this reaction does not mean that water is wanted to quench the thirst. Mokugen means dizziness. Dizziness accompanied by dryness of the mouth is caused by fever. Shoyobyo is a Netsu-sho (fever) somewhere in between Hyo-sho and Ri-sho and is also called Hangaihanri-sho. In addition to the reactions mentioned above, Shoyobyo has the reactions of Kyomankyotsushinhan (pain from pressure in the chest), coughing, palpitation of the heart, fast breathing (difficulty in breathing), nausea, vomiting, and a lack of appetite.

Yomeibyo

When Shoyobyo turns into Ri-sho, it becomes Yomeibyo (yang ming illness). In the Shokan theory, Yomeibyo is explained as a congestion of the stomach and intestines. Therefore, Yomeibyo tends to be characterized by constipation and Fukuman (fullness of the abdomen). Using Fukushin (determination by means of probing the abdomen), a feeling of fullness in the abdomen can be proved. However, even if a person has constipation and Fukuman, he may not have a feeling of congestion in the abdomen. That is, he has Fukuman resulting from Kyoman* or Fukuman resulting from water in the abdomen; for example, Fukuman resulting from cancer, hardening of the liver, and tuberculosis, peritonitis do not generally belong to Yomeibyo.

While Taiyobyo is Hyo-sho, this Yomeibyo is Ri-sho. Yomeibyo is mainly treated by the herbalist with Jokitorui and Byakkoto.

Taiinbyo

In the Shokan theory, Taiinbyo (big yin illness) is

explained as follows: "The reactions of Taiinbyo are Fukuman, vomiting, a lack of purging of the bowels, heavy urination, and sometimes pains in the stomach. If purging of the bowels is attempted, it always ends up with a hardening under the chest."

Fukuman caused by Taiinbyo is kyo and is different from jitsu resulting from Yomeibyo; in addition, Taiinbyo causes vomiting and diarrhea and at times causes a stomachache. When this happens, the pulse is weak and there is no vitality. If this Kyo-sho is misjudged as Jitsu-sho, the region below the heart hardens.

Taiinbyo sometimes results from a misjudgment of Taiyobyo involving the purging of the bowels with a laxative. A person who has a weak stomach and intestines originally may show reactions of Taiinbyo in the early stages of the condition.

Taiinbyo is Rikankyo-sho; and for treatment, herbals containing *Zingiber* (Kankyo)— such as Shakuyakuto (cinnamon bark-*Paeonia* brew), Ninjinto (ginseng brew), Shigyakuto*, and Shinbuto — are used by the herbalist.

Shoinbyo

A person with a delicate constitution or an old person is likely to show Shoinbyo (little yin illness) from the early stages of his condition. Shoinbyo is either Hyo or ri of Kan-sho (cold). In the Shokan theory, it is explained as follows: "Shoinbyo accompanies a weak pulse and the desire to lie down constantly."

Shoinbyo does not cause pain particularly, but stamina is gone; and it makes a person want to lie down. The pulse is also weak; it indicates a deterioration of vitality. In addition, even if the body temperature rises in Shoinbyo, the person's urine is thin, his appetite is good, and his taste for food does not change in many cases. When he is Hyokan-sho, his body aches, he has a headache and chill, and his feet grow cold. When he is Rikan-sho, he has a stomachache, diarrhea, constipation, pressure in the chest, and a large amount of urination.

For treatment of Hyokan reactions, the herbalist will use Maobushikangoto (*Ephedra-Laquiritia* brew) and Maosaishinbushito (*Ephedra-Asarum* brew). For Rikan-sho, Shinbuto or Shigyakuto* is used.

TENZOKU, TENNYU, HEIBYO, GOBYO

Sho is not unchangeable; rather, conditions tend to change. Taiyobyo at the beginning might become Shoyobyo, and later might become Yomeibyo. In some cases, Taiyobyo may become Ketsuinbyo.

Tenzoku means that when one illness (e.g., Taiyobyo) turns into a second illness (e.g., Yomeibyo), the first does not change into Yomeibyo (in this example) completely—some of the reactions of Taiyobyo remain.

If Taiyobyo changes completely into Yomeibyo, then the change is Tennyu.

When Tenzoku occurs, it may be said that the two illnesses are Heibyo (parallel condition). For example, when Tenzoku occurs between Taiyobyo and Yomeibyo, the change becomes the Heibyo of Taiyobyo and Yomeibyo. In this case, Taiyobyo is treated fisrt by the herbalist, and then Yomeibyo.

Gobyo differs from Heibyo in that the person becomes ill with two yangs or even three yangs at the same time; for instance, Taiyobyo-Shoyobyo or Taiyobyo-Yomeibyo or Taiyobyo-Shoyobyo-Yomeibyo.

For treatment in the case of Gobyo with Taiyobyo and Shoyobyo, the herbalist will treat for Shoyobyo; in the case of Gobyo with Taiyobyo and Yomeibyo he will treat for Taiyobyo; in the case of Gobyo with the three yangs, he will use Shosiakoto (Little *Bupleurum* brew) if the Sho for Shoyobyo is predominant, and he will use Byakkoto if the Sho for Yomeibyo is predominant.

KAIBYO

Sometimes, as a result of the wrong type of treatment and for other reasons, Sho breaks down and can no longer be determined correctly. This situation is called Kaiyobyo. For example, if Keishito (cinnamon bark brew) has been administered to bring on perspiration in Taibyo, excessive perspiration will occur, and even before Taiyobyo can be cured, it will already have become partially Shoinbyo. Although it is no longer Taiyobyo, it cannot yet be called Shoinbyo either since the Sho has not completely become Yin-sho. Hence it is called Kaibyo.

PART 2:

Applications of the Herbal Way

NOTE: All the herbal compositions described
herein are to be used only on the advice
and suggestion of a herbalist.

RESPIRATORY CONDITIONS

1. Cold
2. Cough, bronchitis
3. Asthma (bronchial asthma)
4. Cardiac asthma & hoarse voice
5. Dry cough
6. Hemoptysis, bloody phlegm
7. Tubercular cough, whooping cough
8. Tuberculosis
9. Pleurisy

1. Cold

Herbals of choice are

Kakkonto
Kakkontokashinisenkyu
Saikokeishito
Maoto
Shosaikoto

Kakkonto

Fever and inflammation (swelling, pain) generally

are manifestations of the body's resistance to the cause of an internal disorder. Therefore, simple removal of fever or inflammation without destroying the cause of the underlying condition will result in weakening the very resistance. Thus a person may be able to lower his body temperature rapidly by taking a medicine, but his physical condition may deteriorate as a result.

Kakkonto is a herbal that has been modernized from a formula known to early Oriental herbalists. It can remove fever or inflammation as it strengthens the body's resistance to the cause of the condition.

Conditions for which the herbal is effective: colds, coryza, ozena, tonsillitis, conjunctivitis, mastitis, stiff shoulders, neuralgia, migraine. Also for the general conditions of headache, fever, chill, loss of natural perspiration, stiff neck, stiff shoulders, or stiff back, and/or a person with diarrhea.

Selection. For the use of this herb in colds, details are given under Maoto.

For a person with a stiff neck and stiffness throughout the back, this herbal is effective. Kamishoyosan, Daisaikotokyodaio, and Hangebyakujutsutenmato are helpful for those with stiff shoulders.

For a person with similar trouble caused by high blood pressure, one of the following herbals is used: Orengedokuto, Kumibinroto, or Sanoshashinto.

For a person with physiological disorders (vague bodily symptoms difficult to diagnose), either Keishibukeryoganryo or Rokishakuyakusanryo is used.

For a person with an obesity disorder, Daisaikoto or Bofutsushosanryo is used.

To reduce fever in cases of mastitis and tonsillitis, Kakkonto is effective.

Ozena is very unpleasant for it causes one's nose to plug up, excretion of nasal pus, loss of the sense of smell, headache, loss of memory, loss of sleep from irritation, and fatigue. In Japan, it affects many students who are preparing for entrance examinations. The cause of ozena has not been established, but the general consensus is that the cause is related to the physical consequences of stress and nervousness.

Kakkontokashinisenkyu is a new Oriental herbal for internal use; it should be tried first by a person with ozena. It has been proved in many cases to make one feel better and to clear the nose after a few days of use, even in a person with years of suffering or with recurrence after an operation.

Conditions for which the herbal is effective: ozena, chronic inflammation of the nose, clogging of the nose.

Selection. This herb is extremely effective for ozena, inflammation of the nose, and clogging of the nose: After three to five days of use improvement will be noticed.

For a heavy secretion of nasal pus, a combination of Kakkontokashinisenkyu and Kikyosekko is indicated.

For a chronic and stubborn case having a little success by taking Kakkontokashinisenkyu alone, Noza C alone or a combination of Noza C and Kakkontokashinisenkyu is effective.

For headache caused by a light ailment such an inflammation of the nose or clogging of the nose, Kakkonto may also be used.

For a person with thin nasal pus, Shoseiryuto may be used.

For an infant with clogging of the nose that makes it difficult to nurse or to feed from a bottle, Maoto is the most effective herbal.

When a cold is aggravated, it cannot be cured only by lowering the temperature or stopping the cough. It must also be treated with a herbal that will add physical stamina. Saikokeishito is very effective for this purpose. This herbal contains Keishi (cinnamon bark), which has the effect of calming the nerves; Saiko (*Bupleurum*), which strengthens the stomach and intestines and adds Ninjin (Korean variety of ginseng), which strengthens the stomach and intestines and adds physical stamina; and Shakuyaku (*Paeonia, Zingiber, Glycyrrhiza,* and *Zizyphus*), which stops pain and spasm. Its multiple effects are good for the following conditions as well as some of the unpleasant subjective reactions that a woman in her menopause may suffer over a long period of time.

Conditions for which the herbal is effective: colds, pleurisy. For a person with natural perspiration, slight fever accompanied by chills, feeling of oppression in the chest or at the side of the abdomen (in the vicinity of the liver), headache, pain in the chest, nausea, severe abdominal pain, and loss of appetite.

Selection. For a person who suffers aggravation of colds over a long period without signs of improvement, having a slight fever or night sweating, Saikokeishito or Shosaikoto is called for.

In most cases of pleurisy, Saikokeishito or Shosaikoto is effective. If pleurisy is accompanied by pain in the chest or by hydrothorax, Saikanto is the herbal of choice. For a person with an excellent physique and a wide chest who has constipation during pleurisy, Daisaikoto may be used. For a person with a similar build who does not have constipation, Daisaikotokyodaio is recommended.

For a woman during menopause who is bothered by unpleasant emotional reactions for which Saikokeishito is effective (see above), which herbal is recommended.

Maoto

In selecting a herbal for a cold it is important to understand that the recommended herbal differs depending on whether the person has natural perspiration. Maoto is effective when there is a high fever and chills without perspiration or when there is a severe reaction of bodily aches and aching joints. Also, this herb is effective for an infant who has a stopped-up nose and cannot drink milk. When there is a high fever, this herb should be taken with hot water and the person should go to bed; then the body will perspire comfortably and the fever will go down as a result.

Conditions for which the herbal is effective: colds, bronchial asthma, sniffles, stopped-up-nose in an infant. For a person without natural perspiration in spite of high fever and chills, having bodily aches and aching joints. For a person with coughs or asthma.

Selection. This herb is suitable for a cold that may develop complications and require treatment. Please refer to Saikokeishito, above. For a general cold with fever and without perspiration, this herb is indicated. For a person with mild fever and lack of appetite after three or four days of the condition, one of the following may be selected: Shosaikoto, Saikokeishikankyoto, Saikokeishikankyoto, or Hochuekkito.

For a person who coughs, Shoseiryuto may be used.

For an aged person with debility, one of the following is indicated: Kososan, Deishito, Mashininganryo.

For a person with influenza, whose legs and hips ache, Maoto is effective.

At the upper part of the body cavity lie the lungs, heart, stomach, liver, pancreas and other vital organs. When there is a heavy, oppressive, painful, constricted feeling in this vicinity, it is called "oppression of the chest" in Oriental herbalism. If the above organs are weak and a person has a poor physique with a narrow chest, he is said to have scrofulosis (tuberculosis of the lymph glands). Shosaikoto is the herbal used to improve physical characteristics in this case; it is modernized from the herbal Shosankoto, which long was used to remove the oppression in the chest and to improve scrofulosis.

Conditions for which the herbal is effective: chest conditions, improvement of physical stamina after dissipating conditions such as scrofulosis, pleurisy, anemia, gastroenteritis, kidney troubles, colds, bronchitis, bronchial asthma. For a person with oppression in the chest or along the side of the abdomen, slight fever, fatigue, fever and chill alternating, loss of appetite, coating on the tongue, nausea, feeling of vomiting, and cough.

Selection. In general, this herb is very effective for an adult or a child with scrofulosis. Saikoseikanto is also effective.

For an infant with a nervous disorder, the herbal of choice is Shokenchuto or a combination of Shosaikoto with Shokenchuto.

For a person with soft bowel movements, Ninjinto is used.

Shosaikoto is a basic among Oriental herbs and is frequently combined with other herbs in order to improve their physical characteristics.

2. Cough, Bronchitis

Herbals of choice are

Shoseiryuto
Shosaikoto (see page 52)
Bakumonto

Shoseiryuto

If a person does not cough up phlegm while he has bronchial catarrh, his condition is not serious; but if it progresses, light watery phlegm will show up. The treatment is to relieve the inflammation of the lungs and bronchial tubes and to remove mucus. Shoseiryuto is a new Oriental herbal that removes unnecessary water from the body, removes mucus, and stops coughing.

Conditions for which the herbal is effective: bronchitis, bronchial asthma, colds, and kidney trouble. For decreased urination after fever symptoms, for oppression of the chest, and when there is a feeling of water stagnating in the stomach. For a person who coughs with much phlegm accompanied by stridor. For a person with rhinitis draining much nasal mucus, or with hypersecretion such as an eye condition in which copious tears flow.

Selection. For a person coughing from a cold or bronchitis or coughing up phlegm, Shoseiryuto is indicated.

For a person who has thick phlegm, Bakumonto is used.

For a person with dry cough, Hangekobokuto is recommended.

For a person with chronic asthma, the herbalist uses Shinpito or a combination of either Shoseiryuto or

Hangekobokuto with either Shinpito or Daisaikoto, depending on the person's physical characteristics.

For a person with a weak constitution such as anemia or with a cold constitution, Tyokankyomishaingeninto is the herbal of choice.

For a person with coughing from tuberculosis, either Bakumonto or Ninjinyoeito is used.

For a person with asthma, Shoseiryuto is used, but Shinpito may also be used.

Bakumonto

There are various kinds of coughing: dry cough without phlegm, cough with a lot of thin phlegm that clears easily, and cough with sticky and hard-to-clear phlegm. Bakumonto is a new Oriental herbal that clears phlegm, stops stubborn coughs, nourishes the body, and increases physical stamina so that it is effective for a chronic cough or tubercular cough as well as for an old person or a weak person.

Conditions for which the herbal is effective: bronchitis, bronchial asthma, cough due to chest ailment. For a person whose face turns red when heaving up in order to cough strongly. In general, the phlegm is sticky but of small amount, is difficult to cough up, and often is accompanied by blood. For a person with hot fits, thirst, and a feeling of an obstructing foreign material in the throat.

Selection. When a person coughs too severely, his trachea is damaged and bloody phlegm is spit out. Use of Bakumonto in this case is indicated.

For cough from a chest ailment such as tuberculosis, Bakumonto is effective if it is combined with one of the following: Shosaikoto, Hochuekkito, or Saikokeishikankyoto, depending on the reactions.

For whooping cough, Bakumonto is often effective.

3. Asthma (Bronchial Asthma)

Herbals of choice are

Shoseiryuto (see page 53)
Shinpito
Makyokansekito

Shinpito

In most cases, asthma and bronchitis become chronic, and it is necessary to take modern medicines for a long period. But some of these medicines that stop asthmatic seizure and cough have side effects or are habit-forming and harmful to the stomach and intestines. Shinpito is a new Oriental herbal that stops asthmatic coughing and, in addition, contains a herb that strengthens the liver and maintains a healthy stomach as well as a herb that calms the nerves; thus Shinpito is suitable for a long period of continuous usage rather than only for a temporary effect. Therefore, a person can receive treatment as he rebuilds his physical stamina. As the person continues taking this herbal, the number of fits gradually lessens.

Conditions for which the herbal is effective: bronchitis, bronchial asthma. For a person whose condition has become chronic and who has difficulty breathing during coughing seizures.

Selection. In cases of bronchial asthma, this herb is intended as a treatment for gradual recovery by continuous usage over a long period rather than for temporary relief from coughing spells. To stop coughing spells, Makyokansekito is used. As a special treatment for asthma, there are many instances where a person has cured himself of the core of the condition by taking a combination of Hangekobokuto and Shosaikoto, if he is scrofulous, or by taking a combination of Hangekobokuto and Daisaikoto if he is healthy and of strong constitution.

For a person with a delicate, weak, constitution or for an aged person, Ryokankyomishingeninto may do the work.

For a child with asthma, Makyokansekito is indicated.

Please refer to the "Selection" section of Makyokansekito for other usages.

Makyokansekito

Asthmatic convulsion is very painful and is so violent that it can easily upset a person who has to nurse the patient. Often narcotics or powerful medicines are given in order to stop the convulsion; these medicines may seem effective at first, but they are addictive and produce side effects, and they often become harmful if used without caution. Oriental herbals have no side effects. Makyokansekito is a modern extract of Oriental herbs in tablet form that stops convulsions and is effective for the treatment of asthma.

Conditions for which the herbal is effective: bronchitis, bronchial asthma. For a person with severe coughs, perspiration in the head during convulsions accompanied by stridor, and excessive thirst.

Selection. This herb is effective for easing difficult breathing and stopping convulsions of asthma and is also effective for infantile asthma. Better effect may be obtained by combining this herbal with Shosaikoto. (For further detail, please refer to the "Selection" section of Shinpito, above.) For asthma, Makyokansekito is taken daily in a cup of hot water, with sugar added for a child, and given to the person a little at a time as convulsions occur. It quenches the person's thirst and reduces the pain.

4. Cardiac Asthma and Hoarse Voice

The herbal of choice is Hangekobokuto

Hangekobokuto

There are many people who feel tired from the very core, feel uneasy, sleep very lightly, have fast palpitations, and feel like vomiting because of a weak stomach and intestines. Modern doctors may treat them very lightly by saying, "It is only because of nervousness." Hangekobokuto is a modern Oriental herbal that is effective for those complex nervous disorders and that strengthens the stomach and the intestines.

Conditions for which the herbal is effective: neurasthenia, phobia, neurosis, insomnia, menopausal neurosis, nervous headache, bronchitis, bronchial asthma, hoarse voice, coughing spell, weak stomach, morning sickness, vomiting, nervous stricture of the esophagus, edema.

For a person who feels constantly uneasy, feels congested from the throat down to the chest, feels full in the stomach, and has generally poor digestive function, nausea, and vomiting.

Selection. In general, this herb relieves nausea and vomiting and removes the feeling of a thread caught in the throat. For a person with vomiting due to acute gastritis, the herbalist uses either Goreisan or Orento. For a chronic case, Hangeshashinto or Ninjinto is indicated. For violent vomiting due to acute gastritis, Goshuyuto is indicated.

Morning sickness calls for Hangekobokuto or one of the following: Shohangekabukuryoto, Tokishakuyakusanryo, Hangeshashinto, or Rikkunshinto.

Hangekobokuto is effective for cardiac asthma, but also recommended is a combination of Hangekobokuto with Goshakusan or Mokuboito, depending on the symptoms.

5. Dry Cough

The herbal of choice is Saikokeishikankyoto

Saikokeishikankyoto

When weakness is added to conditions originating in the respiratory organs, the heart, and the liver, a person may change mentally also and be inclined toward neurasthenia. In Oriental herbalism, determination of which herb to take depends on how weak a patient has become. Saikokeishikankyoto is used when a patient is considerably weakened physically and mentally.

Conditions for which the herbal is effective: cold, cardiac weakness, chest disorders, lack of physical stamina after dissipatory illness such as liver ailment, anemia, neurasthenia, amnesia, menopausal neurosis. For a person in run-down condition who shows poor complexion, slight fever, head perspiration, night sweating, loss of appetite, awareness of throbbing in the chest or around the navel, insomnia caused by neurasthenic tendency, tendency to have soft bowel movements, reduced amount of urination, dryness inside the mouth, and dry cough.

Selection. In cases of heart disease and cardiac weakness, when the person has lost stamina and experiences neurasthenic tendency, Saikokeishikankyoto or Keishikaryukotsuboreito is used.

For a person with constipation but without a rundown condition, Saikokaryukotsuboreito is used.

For a person with anemia or a cold constitution, either Tokishakuyakusanryo or Ryokyojutsukanto is used.

For a person with a weak heart from obesity, Bofutsushosanryo is used.

For a person with irregular but fast palpitation, Shakanzoto is used.

For a person with a headache and dizziness when standing up, Reikeijutsukanto is used.

For a person with stridor, Mokuboito is used.

For a person with beriberi, Kumibinroto is used.

6. Hemoptysis, Bloody Phlegm

Herbals of choice are

Bakumonto (see page 54)
Orengedokuto
Shakanzoto

Orengedokuto (To be used only under a medical doctor's supervision)

Both Oren and Obaku*, which are raw materials for Oriental herbs, contain beriberine and are effective for high blood pressure and arteriosclerosis. They will stop various kinds of bleeding by relaxing the abnormal contraction of the capillary vessels. In addition, they are effective for nervous disorders such as hot fits and insomnia. Both of these herbs are very bitter in its original form, but Orengedokuto is prepared from these two principal herbs in a way that makes it easier to drink and more effective.

Conditions for which the herbal is effective: gastritis, hangover, stomatitis, nervous disorders, high blood pressure, insomnia due to high blood pressure, vomiting of blood, discharge of blood, nose bleeding. For a person who has hot fits, stiff shoulders, or a choked stomach, and for a person who has constipation with soft stools, or has blood-shot eyes.

Selection. Bleeding: For a nervous person who bleeds for various reasons, this herb is useful.

For a person with rectal bleeding and constipation, Sanoshashinto is used.

For a person with hemoptysis, Shosaikoto in combination with Orengedokuto is indicated.

For a weak person with atonic bleeding, Hochuekkito is indicated.

For an anemic person after prolonged bleeding, Kyukikyogaito is used.

For a person of reddish dark skin with constipation and bleeding from hemorrhoids, the herbalist uses Daiobotanpito.

For a person with itchy eczema and severe hot fits, a combination of Orengedokuto and Shimotsuto is used to give good results.

Shakanzoto

Conditions for which the herbal is effective: cardiac neurosis, valvular disease of the heart, cough with bloody phlegm, breathing difficulty due to Graves' disease. For a person with bad complexion, anemia, arrhythmia, palpitation, shortness of breath, tendency to constipate, and slight fever.

NOTE: This herb is unsuitable for a person who has a weak stomach and diarrhea.

7. Tubercular Cough, Whooping Cough

The herbal of choice is Bakumonto (see page 54)

8. Tuberculosis

Herbals of choice are

Hochuekkito
Saikokeishikankyoto (see page 58)
Bakumonto (see page 54)

Hochuekkito

Many people benefit little no matter how long they patiently take hormone tablets. It appears that the cause lies in the fact that functional defects of the stomach and intestines or the liver prevent proper absorption of the hormone. Hochuekkito is an Oriental herbal in tablet form based primarily on Chosen Ninjin (Korean variety of ginseng), which prepares the receiving systems as it builds up the stomach and intestines or the liver and nourishes the body.

Conditions for which the herbal is effective: physical debility, loss of physical stamina due to tuberculosis or illness, scrofula, loss of weight in summer, anemia, weak stomach, low blood pressure, hemorrhoids, proctocele. For a person with poorly functioning stomach and intestines accompanied by feeling of constant fatigue. For a person with headache, chills, night sweating, or atonic bleeding.

Selection. In cases of scrofula, weakness, debility, loss of weight, and tubercular physique, Hochuekkito—a famous body-building and nourishing product—is effective in building body strength and stamina quickly.

For a person with scrofula, with Hochuekkito use Shokenchuto, Shosaikoto, or Saikoseikanto.

For a person with debility due to a tubercular physique or illness, use Hochuekkito, Saikokeishikankyoto, Juzentaihoto, or Ninjinyoeito.

For a person who has had a major operation and is very weak mentally and physically, Juzentaihoto may be more effective than Hochuekkito.

9. Pleurisy

The herbals of choice are

Saikokeishito (see page 50)
Shosaikoto (see page 52)

DIGESTIVE CONDITIONS

1. Stomachache, stomach cramp, heartburn, gastritis
2. Gastroptosis, gastric atony, gastric dilation
3. Stomach ulcer, duodenal ulcer
4. Stomach neurosis
5. Inveterate dyspepsia (diarrhea, loose bowels, stomachache, vomiting and purging)
6. Acute gastroenteritis, hangover
7. Enteritis, loose bowels with gripping pain
8. Poor appetite
9. Nervous esophagostenosis (stricture of the throat)
10. Hiccups
11. Nausea, vomiting
12. Constipation
13. Liver trouble
14. Jaundice, cholecystitis, cholelithiasis
15. Appendicitis
16. Peritonitis
17. Stomatitis

1. Stomachache, Stomach Cramp, Heartburn, Gastritis

Herbals of choice are

Anchusanryo
Orengedokuto (see page 59)
Heisanryo

Anchusanryo

Recently, gastroenteric conditions have been increasing in civilized countries; but in order to cure them at the root of the cause, it is of no use to take habitually a medicine that kills the pain temporarily. Especially for neurogastroenteric disorders, which account for more than 50 percent of all gastroenteric patients, it is necessary to control the abnormal reactions of the nerves instead of using only medicines for stopping the pain or the heartburn. Anchusanryo is a modern Oriental herb that works quickly on gastroenteric conditions accompanied by nervousness and a cold constitution.

Conditions for which the herbal is effective: gastroenteritis, gastritis, acid dyspepsia (pyrosis), stomachache due to ulcer. For persons with stomachache and pyrosis who have a cold constitution and are nervous.

Selection. For gastritis (pyrosis, stomachache), gastric dilation: Anchusanryo is the best remedy. When stomachache is severe, this herb is combined with Saikokeishito. When stomachache is caused by overeating, Heisanryo is used.

For a person with excess fat who suffers from dyspepsia, Bofutsushosanryo is recommended.

For other cases refer to Orengedokuto, Daisaikoto, Goshakusan, Shakuyakukuanzoto* and Bukuryoin.

There are commercial medicines for treatment of the stomach that are only temporarily effective, and which become habit forming, resulting in the need to take increasing amounts. Heisanryo is an aromatic, vegetative digestive aid thoughtfully recommended in place of sodium bicarbonate or scopolia extract (powerful medicine). It increases appetite and digestion and is effective for overeating or disorders caused by water-poisoning. There is no problem of side effects or addiction to this herbal.

Conditions for which the herbal is effective: gastritis, atony of the stomach, gastric dilation, stomatitis. For a person with stomachache caused by indigestion, other abdominal pain, loss of appetite, or growling of the stomach after meals which is accompanied by diarrhea.

Selection. This herb is effective for loss of appetite following overeating or food-poisoning. Shosaikoto is frequently used also. The herbal is chosen depending on the cause, such as disorder of the stomach and intestines or the liver, debility of the entire body, and nervousness. Besides these herbals, for loss of appetite caused by chronic gastroenteric disorder, the herbalist uses one of the following: Hangeshashinto, Rikkunshito, Orento, Ninjinto, or Bukuryoin.

For disorders originating in the stomach and intestines or the liver, the herbalist chooses one of the following: Shosaikoto, Daisaikoto, or Daisaikotokyodaio.

For lack of appetite due to nervousness, Kososan or Kamishoyosan should be used.

For lack of appetite due to debility, Saikokeishikankyoto, Shokenchuto, or Ninjinyoeito should be administered.

2. Gastroptosis, Gastric Atony, Gastric Dilation

Herbals of choice are

Rikkunshito
Anchusanryo (see page 63)
Hangeshashinto

Rikkunshito

Gastric atony is a condition in which the stomach muscles become weak and the stomach sags down below the navel. These reactions occur in skinny people who have excess water content in the stomach, which causes belching, nausea, loss of appetite, headache, dizziness, etc., all of which are nervous disorders. Rikkunshito removes unnecessary water in the stomach, increases digestive and absorptive power, and is effective in adding weight in a skinny person.

Conditions for which the herbal is effective: gastric atony, dilation of the stomach, gastritis, nervous disorder of the stomach, morning sickness, lack of appetite in a weak child. For a person with anemia, cold constitution, oppression of the stomach, a tendency to have soft bowel movements, and who is easily fatigued.

Selection. For gastric atony and nervous disorder of the stomach, generally this herbal is most widely used. A person will not be conscious of his weak stomach after continuous use. Also, Hangeshashinto may be used.

In addition to these herbs, Juzentaihoto or Hochuekkito is effective for a skinny person who loses weight.

For a person with chronic diarrhea, the herbalist uses Ninjinto.

For a person with stomachache or heartburn, the herbalist uses Anchusanryo.

For a person with severe headache caused by stagnation of water in the stomach, the herbalist uses Hangebyakujutsutenmato or Bukuryoin.

For a very nervous female with stomach trouble, the herbalist uses Kamishoyosan.

Hangeshashinto

For a person who constantly suffers from diarrhea or soft bowel movements and seems unable to sustain any nourishment in his body, or for a person who alternates between diarrhea and constipation, treatment takes time and consequently he suffers long. The characteristic common reactions of this condition are that his stomach feels stuffy and growls and that he feels uneasy. Hangeshashinto is an Oriental herbal in tablet form that removes stuffiness in the stomach, controls bowel movements, and restores physical stamina.

Conditions for which the herbal is effective: acute or chronic catarrh of the stomach and intestines, fermentative diarrhea, indigestion, stomatitis, and morning sickness. For a person with stuffy stomach who is nauseous and feels like vomiting.

For a person with loss of appetite and coated tongue who feels water stagnating in the stomach accompanied by growling and who eventually has diarrhea.

For a person with soft bowel movements or liquid stool.

Selection. In cases of chronic gastroenteritis (diarrhea, stomachache, indigestion), this herbal is very effective. Also, Rikkunshito may be used. Besides these herbals, Anchusanryo may be used if a person has heartburn.

For infantile gastoenteric disorders, either Shokenchuto or Saikoseikanto is recommended.

The causes of loss of appetite are rather complex. Depending on the physical characteristics, the herbalist will use one of the following: Shosaikoto, Daisaikoto, Hangekobokuto, Daisaikotokyodaio, or Bukuryion.

For a person with gastroenteritis due to overeating, he will use Heisanryo.

For a person with a cold constitution, he will use Goshakusan.

For chronic diarrhea, he will use either Shinbutc or Ninjinto.

3. Stomach Ulcer, Duodenal Ulcer

Herbals of choice are

Anchusanryo (see page 63)
Hangeshashinto (see page 66)
Rikkunshito (see page 65)

4. Stomach Neurosis

Herbals of choice are

Rikkunshito (see page 65)
Hangeshashinto (see page 66)

5. Inveterate Dyspepsia (Diarrhea, Loose Bowels, Stomachache, Vomiting and Purging)

Herbals of choice are

Hangeshashinto (see page 66)
Anchusanryo (see page 63)
Heisanryo (see page 64)
Rikukunshito (see page 65)

6. Acute Gastroenteritis, Hangover

The herbal of choice is Orengedokuto (see page 59)

7. Enteritis, Loose Bowels with Gripping Pain

The herbal of choice is Keishikashakuyakuto*

*Keishikashakuyakuto**

Conditions for which the herbal is effective: loose bowels with gripping pain, enteritis, chronic appendicitis, chronic peritonitis. For a person with a feeling of a full stomach and abdominal pain accompanied by diarrhea or constipation or vomiting.

NOTE: This herbal is effective for severe abdominal pain and is used in combination with Daio, if constipation is present.

8. Poor Appetite

Herbals of choice are

Hangeshashinto (see page 66)
Heisanryo (see page 64)
Shosaikoto (see page 52)
Rikkunshito (see page 65)

9. Nervous Esophagostenosis (Stricture of the Throat)

The herbal of choice is Hangekobokuto (see page 57)

10. Hiccups

The herbal of choice is Goshuyuto

Goshuyuto

Conditions for which the herbal is effective: spastic headache, vomiting, headache on one side, hiccups. For a person with a cold constitution accompanied by headache, oppressions of the stomach, nausea, or vomiting.

NOTE: This herb is suitable for severe reactions of the above kinds of conditions.

11. Nausea, Vomiting

Herbals of choice are

Hangekobokuto (see page 57)
Hangeshashinto (see page 66)

12. Constipation

Herbals of choice are

Mashininganryo
Sanoshashinto
Daisaikoto

Mashininganryo

Habitual constipation is the cause of headache, hot fits, high blood pressure, and poor texture of the skin; it also quickens the aging process of the body. If a strong laxative is used for constipation, the physical stamina is lost; therefore, care should be taken. Ideally, bowel movement should occur once or twice a day with ease. Mashininganryo is a mild laxative appropriate even for a weakened person or an aged person. About ten hours after taking this herb, a person will have an easy bowel movement. However, depending on the individual, effectiveness varies; therefore each person should arrive at his own proper dosage through experience.

Conditions for which the herbal is effective: habitual constipation, acute constipation, constipation after illness, hemorrhoids with constipation, atrophied kidney.

Selection. For constipation. This herbal is used even for an aged person or a child. For a person with constipation who has physical stamina and feels good after each bowel movement, the herbalist uses one of the following: Kumibinroto, Sanoshashinto, Daisaikoto, Togakujokito, Bofutsushosanryo, or Daiobotanpito, depending on the physical characteristics. If there is no result, add Daio to whatever herbal is being used. For a person with dry bowel movements or with bowel movements that turn soft after the first hard stool, one of the following will strengthen the intestines: Shokenchuto, Shosaikoto, Hangeshashinto, or Daijokito. It is important to watch one's food consumption when constipated; eat many more vegetables and seaweeds.

Sanoshashinto

The high blood pressure of a person who has hot fits, a red face, a thick short neck, and a tendency toward apoplexy, is called red high blood pressure. That of a person who is of a thin type and pale, is called white high blood pressure. Their physical characteristics are completely different, and thus different Oriental herbals are used for each type. Sanoshashinto is an herbal with outstanding effectiveness for a person with red high blood pressure who has severe constipation. Similar to Orengedokuto, this herbal has Oren and Obaku* as the principal ingredients and combined with Daiois laxative. It is very effective for high blood pressure and for neurasthenia and constipation.

Conditions for which the herbal is effective: high blood pressure, arteriosclerosis, cerebral hemorrhage, insomnia due to high blood pressure, vomiting of blood, discharge of blood, nose bleed, and habitual constipation.

Selection. For a person with hot fits accompanied by mental uneasiness, a choked feeling in the stomach, or severe constipation accompanied by mental uneasiness, the herbalist uses Sanoshashinto.

For a woman with the above conditions, Togakujokito is effective. Combination of Sanoshashinto with either Daisaikoto or Togakujokito is partially effective.

For a person without constipation Orengedokuto or Yokukansankachinbihange is recommended.

For a person with stiff shoulders and a feeling of fatigue, Kumibinroto is effective.

For a person with constipation and insomnia, Saikokaryukotsuboreito or Daisaikoto is suggested.

For a person with much urination and cold hips, use Hachimiganryo.

For a person who is obese, use Bofutsushosanryo.

Daisaikoto

A person in his prime tends to overwork himself mentally and physically, so that he is liable to suffer from neurasthenia, gastroenteritis, or liver trouble. Also, this is the time when the aging process sets in. A person with a strong physique has a natural tendency to become overconfident about his health and tends to overwork himself until rapid deterioration sets in. Daisaikoto has an excellent effect on acute conditions in this type of person and is used for the following reactions.

Conditions for which the herbal is effective: high blood pressure, arteriosclerosis, hemiplegia, obesity, neurasthenia, gastroenteric disorders, jaundice, cholelithiasis, cholecystisis, habitual constipation, insomnia, impotence, bronchial asthma, hemorrhoids. For a person with oppression of the liver or with tightness around the pit of the stomach that causes pain or oppression of the chest or with tightness of the side of the abdomen accompanied by constipation or loose bowels, along with diarrhea. For a person with tinnitus aurium, stiff shoulders, a feeling of fatigue, or loss of appetite.

Selection. For a person with a strong constitution who has liver trouble accompanied by constipation, use Daisaikoto. For a person with liver trouble without constipation, use Daisaikotokyodaio. For a thin person with a weak liver and constipation, Shosaikoto is the herbal of choice. Saikokeishito is also effective.

For a person with the same reactions who has no constipation, use Shishihakuhito. This herbal is for the improvement of physical characteristics for a middle-aged person or for an elderly person who maintains a strong physique, and is used in many instances with other herbals.

13. Liver Trouble

Herbals of choice are

Daisaikoto (see page 71)
Shosaikoto (see page 52)

14. Jaundice, Cholecystitis, Cholelithiasis

Herbals of choice are

Inchinkoto
Daisaikoto (see page 71)

Inchinkoto

Jaundice plays a significant role in the determination of liver troubles. Even with slight jaundice, a person has a headache and feels fatigued; his skin turns yellow and he is bothered by extreme itchiness. Cholecystitis is caused by contagious germs in a person with cholelithiasis (gallstones) and causes pain, high fever, jaundice, and enlargement of the liver. In either case, early treatment with sufficient care is required. Inchinkoto helps the function of the liver and secretion of bile. This herbal is modernized from the traditional Inchinkoto, which has long been popular for the early treatment of liver and cystic ailments.

Conditions for which the herbal is effective: for those with constant thirst, feeling of oppression of the chest, or constipation, and for those with oppressive pain in the liver area who develop jaundice. Also for hives, cholecystitis, and stomatitis.

Selection. For jaundice and cholecystitis: when the reactions are severe, with constipation, this herb alone is used. As the illness becomes chronic, the herbalist will use a combination of this herbal with Goreisan. For well-built persons with regular bowel movements, the herbalist will use Daisaikoto or a combination of Inchinkoto with Daisaikoto. For those who object to laxatives, Shishihakuhito or Daisaikotokyodaio is used.

In case of cholelithiasis, use Daisaikoto if constipated. Use Shakuyakukanzoto if pain is severe. For those who object to laxatives, Daisaikotokyodaio may be used.

15. Appendicitis

Herbals of choice are

Daiobotanpito
Keishikashakuyakuto* (see page 68)
Choyoto

Daiobotanpito

Conditions for which the herbal is effective: habitual constipation, arteriosclerosis, menoxenia and resulting disorders, menopausal disorders, eczema, urticaria, comedones, swelling with pus, catarrh of the bladder. For a person with oppressive pain of the caecum or constipation, hard stools, purple or dark red skin texture, and a tendency to have blood congestion or bleeding.

NOTE: This herb is very effective for inflammation in the lower half of the body.

Choyoto

Conditions for which the herbal is effective: for a person with acute or chronic pain in the caecum, or for a woman with menostasis.

NOTE: This herb is suitable for chronic pain in the caecum or a movable caecum.

16. Peritonitis

Herbals of choice are

Keishikashakuyakuto* (see page 68)
Daikenchuto

Daikenchuto

Conditions for which the herbal is effective: dilation of the stomach, gastric atony, atonic diarrhea, atonic constipation, chronic peritonitis, abdominal pain. For a person with atonic abdominal wall or atonic stomach and intestines, chills in the abdomen, vomiting, stuffiness in the abdomen, and severe pain in the abdomen as the intestines make peristaltic motion.

NOTE: This herb is prepared for the person whose abdomen is without strength and atonic.

17. Stomatitis

Herbals of choice are

Heisanryo (see page 64)
Orengedokuto (see page 59)

CIRCULATORY CONDITIONS

1. Heart disease, endocarditis, valvular disease of the heart
2. Tachycardia (palpitation)
3. High blood pressure, arteriosclerosis, hemiplegia
4. Low blood pressure, abnormal blood pressure
5. Beriberi

1. Heart Condition, Endocarditis, Valvular Disease of the Heart

Herbals of choice are

Saikokeishikankyoto (see page 58)

Tokishakuyakusanryo
Reikeijutsukanto

Tokishakuyakusanryo

The ovaries and uterus of a woman who suffers from a metabolic disorder of water content, which causes anemia or a cold constitution, will weaken and will cause instability of the autonomic nerves; thus, she presents reactions of various kinds of mental and physical ills and quickens the deteriorations of the aging process. Tokishakuyakusanryo is an excellent Oriental herbal in tablet form that is very effective for delicate female disorders that affect a woman mentally and physically.

Conditions for which the herbal is effective: menoxenia, pain during menstruation, menopausal nervous disorder, morning sickness, cardiac weakness, anemia, abnormal blood pressure, kidney disease, anemia caused by childbirth or abortion, hemorrhoids, proctocele, comedones, blemishes. For a person with anemia or a cold constitution accompanied by a weak stomach and intestines, who has dark circles around the eyes and who is easily fatigued, feels heavy in the head, feels dizzy, has stiff shoulders, and has rapid palpitation of the heart. For a person with frequent but small amounts of urination, and with constant thirst. For a person with a cold constitution accompanied by an oppressive feeling of pain in the abdomen. For a person who easily suffers frostbite.

Selection. Tokishakuyakusanryo is the typical herb for female disorders, and it is effective for the above listed diseases.

For a person with a weak stomach and intestines, a

combination of Tokishakuyakusanryo and Shosaikoto is suggested.

For physiological disorders, refer to the "Selection" section of Keishibukeryoganryo, page 97.

For menopause, refer to Togakujokito, page 107.

For a cold constitution, Tokishakuyakusanryo is effective, as are the following: Keishibukeryoganryo, Shokenchuto, Togakujokito, Tokushigyakukagokyoto and Hachimiganryo.

Reikeijutsukanto

Autonomic nervousness has recently become a problem. It causes dizziness, unsteadiness of the body, headache all year round, and causes one to become very sensitive; these reactions affect the internal organs and bring out various nervous disorders. In Oriental herbalism, the relationship between the nerves and the internal organs has been considered very important since early days, and Reikeijutsukanto has been used for those reactions. Reikeijutsukanto is a modern herbal in tablet form.

Conditions for which the herbal is effective: nervous disorders, palpitation caused by nervousness, tinnitus aurium, insomnia, congestion of the blood, abnormal blood pressure, weak heart, kidney trouble. For a person who becomes dizzy on standing up, is often dizzy, has fast palpitations, hot fits accompanied by headache, flushed face, anemia, frequent but small amounts of urination, or dry mouth and lips.

Selection. For dizziness, dizziness on standing, heavy-headedness: to relieve these reactions in a person with low blood pressure, Meniere's disease, or anemia, this herbal is most effective. Also for a person with chronic

77

headache that has been bothering him for years, this herb is effective.

For a woman with physiological disorders or menopause, the herbalist will use either Keishibukeryoganryo or Tokishakuyakusanryo.

For a person with nervous disorder, the herbalist will use Kososan, Saikokaryukotsuboreito or Keishikaryukotsuboreito. Also refer to the "Selection" section of Kososan, page 96.

2. Tachycardia (Palpitation)

Herbals of choice are

> Saikokaryukotsuboreito
> Kumibinroto
> Reikeijutsukanto (see page 77)

Saikokaryukotsuboreito

One of the cardinal principles in Oriental herbalism is to use a herbal composition that will be suitable to the constitution, and this principle must not be disregarded for conditions mainly concerning nerves. Saikokaryukotsuboreito is an Oriental herbal that is superbly effective for the following list of conditions. The herb is effective for a youth or a person at his prime who has a history of constipation and neurotic tendency.

Conditions for which the herbal is effective: arteriosclerosis, high blood pressure, neurosis, insomnia, nervous palpitation, menopausal neurosis, infantile crying at night, impotence, kidney disease, cardiac weakness. For a person with nervous uneasiness who frightens easily and has palpitation, severe pain in the chest, dizziness, hot fits, and insomnia, or one who becomes aware of throbbing around the navel, feels tight around

78

the pit of the stomach, is constipated, and has reduced amounts of urination.

Selection. For a person with nervous palpitation causing constipation, Saikokaryukotsuboreito is used. For nervous palpitation without constipation, the herbalist uses Keishikaryukotsuboreito. For a person with palpitation due to beriberi, the herbalist uses Kumibinroto.

For a person with physiological disorders, he uses Keishibukeryoganryo. For a person with palpitation accompanied by dizziness when standing up, the herbalist uses Reikeijutsukanto.

Loss of hair: for a youth with premature baldness, Keishikaryukotsuboreito is recommended.

Kumibinroto

As vitamin pills have become available universally, vitamin B_1 deficiency has decreased tremendously, but there are still many people who drag their feet and tend to tire easily with signs of beriberi and a tendency to constipate. Kumibinroto in such cases is extremely effective and will remove the feeling of fatigue and make one feel physically pleasant. This effectiveness seems to stem from the fact that this herbal promotes the efficient use of vitamins and also helps absorption of nutrients by the intestines. In addition, it is effective for high blood pressure.

Conditions for which the herbal is effective: beriberi, high blood pressure, and arteriosclerosis and ensuing headache. For a person with tachycardia, stiff shoulders, a feeling of fatigue, and a tendency to constipate.

Selection. For a feeling of fatigue (without exhaustion), for a person with dragging feet, constipation, arteriosclerosis, and general fatigue, this herb is used. For a person with bad stomach and intestines who tires easily, the herbalist will use either Daisaikoto or Shosaikoto. For a person with weak constitution or one who is run-down and tires easily, refer to the "Selection" section of Hochuekkito, page 61.

In general this herb is effective for beriberi, but for a person with bad swelling, Eppikajutsuto is more effective.

For a person with cold constitution who has a healthy stomach and intestines, use Goshakusan.

3. High Blood Pressure, Arteriosclerosis, Hemiplegia

Herbals of choice are

Sanoshashinto (see page 70)
Daisaikoto (see page 71)
Yokukansankachinbihange

Yokukansankachinbihange

Palpitation, uneasiness, fear, heavy-headedness, hot fits, dizziness, stiff shoulders, insomnia, and a weary feeling of the whole body—all of these nervous reactions have been complained of not only by neurotic persons but also by persons with high blood pressure, arteriosclerosis, or menopause and by nervous children. Yokukansankachinbihange consists primarily of Kintoko, which contains licorfilyne, a pain-killer, tranquilizer and depressant that calms abnormal excitation of the cerebrum and strengthens the stomach and intestines as well as the liver. Yokukansankachinbihange is made from the essence of nine herbs into tablet form.

Conditions for which the herbal is effective: nervousness (neurosis), menopausal nervousness, insomnia, nervousness caused by high blood pressure or arterio-sclerosis, infantile night crying.

Selection. Applicable to cases of neurosis, neurasthenia, and insomnia, as follows. This herbal is effective for nervousness caused by high blood pressure or abnormal blood pressure. Other herbals such as Orengedokuto, Sanoshashinto, Daisaikoto, and Reikeijutsukanto may be used depending on the physical make-up.

For a person with debility, either Saikokeishikank-yoto or Juzentaihoto is used.

For a person having anxiety with nervousness one of the following will be helpful: Hangekobokuto, Tok-ishakuyakusanryo, Kososan, Kamishoyosan, or Kan-bakutaisoto.

For a child, use Shokenchuto, Kanbakutaisoto, or Saikoseikanto.

For a person with sexual neurosis, the herbalist will choose between Saikokaryukotsuboreito or Keishikaryu-kotsuboreito.

4. Low Blood Pressure, Abnormal Blood Pressure

Herbals of choice are

Juzentaihoto
Tokishakuyakusanryo (see page 76)
Hochuekkito (see page 61)

Juzentaihoto

Juzentaihoto is modernized from the famous Juzen-taihoto, a traditional Oriental herbal for nourishment, robustness, and improvement of physical stamina. This herbal is effective against conditions that severely drain physical stamina, such as tuberculosis or general debility after an operation, or serious conditions of childbirth; it acts by increasing the appetite, the digestive absorptive power, and the recovery from anemia.

Conditions for which the herbal is effective: for thin anemic persons with pale, nonlustrous skin and mucous membranes, or for a person who has no appetite and has grown seriously weak. For a person with the following reactions from debility caused by exhaustive illness (liver trouble, tuberculosis, etc.) or from debility after an operation, after childbirth, and from general prostration: anemia, low blood pressure, feeling of constant fatigue, neurasthenia, gastroenteric debility, gastroptosis.

Selection. In cases of weakness, debility, anemia, loss of weight, night sweating: Juzentaihoto or Hochuekkito is effective for recovery from these reactions following a serious illness, operation, or childbirth. For nervous persons, use Saikokeishikankyoto. For a child with debility, use either Shokenchuto or Saikoseikanto. For a person with a bad liver, use Shosaikoto. For an anemic woman with a cold constitution, use Tokishakuyakusanryo, Tokushigyakukagokyoto or Shimotsuto. For a person who is anemic due to bleeding, use Kyukikyogaito.

For a person with debility and low blood pressure use either Juzentaihoto or Hochuekkito. For an aged person with a cold constitution, use Hachimiganryo.

For a person with low blood pressure causing dizziness when standing up, use Reikeijutsukanto.

For a person with low blood pressure and a weak stomach and intestines, use Hangebyakujutsutenmato.

5. Beriberi

Herbals of choice are

Kumibinroto (see page 79)
Eppikajutsuto

About seventy percent of the body weight consists of water. Water content of the body is supplied by intake of drinks and food and is excreted as perspiration or urine, but if the excretion is interrupted and water is accumulated in the periphery of the body, the whole body swells, or blisters, and eczema with profuse secretion may appear. Eppikajutsuto is a new Oriental herbal that can strengthen the functioning of the kidneys, regulate the flow of urine comfortably, remove the interruption of water secretion rapidly, cure constant thirst, and prevent the supply of overabundant water content.

Conditions for which the herbal is effective: nephritis, nephrosis, eczema, beriberi. For a person with constant thirst, severe edema or blisters, decrease in the amount of urine, or frequent urination, or for a person with profuse secretion.

Selection. For edema (bloating, swelling): when swelling is excessive without debility, the herbalist will use this herbal alone. When the mouth is dry and a little swelling appears, the herbalist will use Goreisan. For an aged person with a cold constitution having swelling he will use Hachimiganryo. For a nervous person with slight swelling, the herbalist will use Hangekobokuto.

For a person with perspiratory disorders that cause the whole body to swell, Boiogito is recommended.

For a person with edema and a bad heart, Nankuboito* is suggested.

Eppikajutsuto is very effective for blisters such as those of chicken pox or eczema with much secretion.

URINATION, GENITAL TROUBLES

1. Nephritis, nephrosis
2. Atrophied kidney
3. Urethritis, cystitis, kidney and bladder stones
4. Abnormal urination (frequent urination, infrequent urination)
5. Edema
6. Loss of vitality, impotence, sexual neurasthenia

1. Nephritis, Nephrosis

Herbals of choice are

Goreisan
Choreito
Tokishakuyakusanryo (see page 76)
Hachimiganryo

Goreisan

There is no decisive cure by modern medical treatment for kidney trouble. If it is acute, it may take one to two months to cure, and if it is chronic, it becomes difficult to cure and is accompanied by high blood pressure or by cardiac weakness. It further develops into nephrosis, atrophied kidneys, and uremia.

Like kidney trouble, acute gastroenteritis which causes vomiting and watery diarrhea is also a disease caused by metabolic interruption of the water content. Goreisan is a product modernized from a traditional Oriental herb for the relief of metabolic interruption of water content.

Conditions for which the herbal is effective: nephritis, nephrosis, catarrh of the bladder, acute gastroenteritis, infantile diarrhea, hangover, sunstroke, jaundice. For a person with a decrease of urine even after a large consumption of water, or for a person with a headache, heavy-headedness, head perspiration, nausea, or feeling of edema.

Selection. For nephritis or nephrosis, Goreisan is most suitable.

For a person weakened by a chronic case, a combination of this herb with Shosaikoto is effective.

For a person with severe swelling, either Eppikajutsuto or Mokuboito may be used.

For a person with neurosis, Saikokaryukotsuboreito is suggested.

For a person having difficulty urinating, the herbalist uses Choreito.

For a person with a cold constitution, the herbalist uses either Tokishakuyakusanryo or Hachimiganryo.

For a person of corpulence, Bofutsushosanryo is recommended.

In cases of hangover and acute gastritis, when the person is vomiting and purging or having a headache, the herbalist uses either Goreisan or Orengedokuto or a combination of the two for immediate effect.

Choreito

It is very uncomfortable to have difficult urination with pain or bleeding. Even if antibiotics may have sterilizing power, they have no capacity to restore the injured urethra or bladder. Consequently, unpleasant reactions remain. A cold constitution or vesical calculi cause these reactions. Choreito is an Oriental herbal in tablet form that removes inflammation while it increases urination comfortably and thus stops pain in a short time.

Conditions for which the herbal is effective: catarrh of the bladder, urethritis, nephritis, nephrosis, difficulty with urination caused by vesical calculi. For a person with thirst accompanied by pain during urination or by difficulty of urination wherein the urine turns red or contains blood, or for a person with edema in the hips or in the lower limbs.

Selection. Choreito is generally effective for urethritis, cystitis, renal calculi, and vesical calculi. For a person with extreme thirst, Goreisan is used. For an old person with cold hips, Hachimiganryo is used. For a person with constipation, Daiobotanpito is used. For a person with urethritis, cystitis, or renal or vesical calculi resulting from bacterial infection, the herbalist uses Ryutanshakanto. For a person with frequent urination, the herbalist will select one of the following: Shokenchuto, Tokishakuyakusanryo, Hachimiganryo, or Ryokojutsukanto. For a person with infrequent urination, the herbalist will select one of the following: Goreisan, Togakujokito, or Choreito.

Hachimiganryo

Withering of the hormone-producing organs and sclerosis of the kidneys, with decreased energy, pain in the hip, and the necessity for frequent urination at night are all part of the aging process. Hachimiganryo, modernized from the famous Hachimigan, is effective for the following conditions for a person over forty years old who needs energy and physical stamina.

Conditions for which the herbal is effective: diabetes, impotence, sciatica, arteriosclerosis, chronic nephritis, nephrosis, atrophied kidney, catarrh of the bladder, edema, menopausal disorder, eczema of the aged, low blood pressure, beriberi after childbirth. For a person

Nervousness is defined as (1) an emotional condition in which emotion becomes excitable; (2) nervous conditions, such as fatigue, insomnia, etc.; and (3) physical conditions such as indigestion, night sweating, etc. Nervousness is so complex a condition that it often is difficult to find the true cause. For example, bed-wetting seems to occur mostly among nervous children. When a child becomes neurotic, his physical growth will be hindered.

Shokenchuto is a new Oriental herb that increases the physical strength and vigor collectively and is effective as well as sweet and easy to take for the following diseases.

Conditions for which the herbal is effective: nervousness, scrofulosis, anemia, crying at night by a baby, gastroenteritis, diarrhea or constipation in an infant, frequent urination, bed-wetting in an infant, and night crying. For a person with a delicate and weak constitution who tires easily, who has hot fits, pain in the abdomen, palpitation, and a cold constitution with hands and legs that are hot, and who urinates frequently in large amounts.

Selection. For infantile neurasthenia, night crying, night fright: Shokenchuto is easy to drink as well as being effective.

For a person especially with a tendency toward constipation, use Saikokaryukotsuboreito.

For an infant who cries violently at night, use Yokukansankachinbihange or Kanbakutaisoto.

For a person with a nervous disorder together with scrofulous physical characteristics, use Saikoseikanto.

Shokenchuto is effective for bed-wetting; also keep in mind that bed-wetting is said to be caused by unful-

89

filled desires, and it is important to remove its cause. Keishikaryukotsuboreito is also effective. For a child with a cold constitution who wets his bed, use either Hachimiganryo or Ryokyojutsukanto.

2. Hemorrhage (Coughing-Up Blood), Vomiting Blood, Nose Bleeding, Bleeding of Hemorrhoids, Bleeding After Childbirth

Herbals of choice are

  Orengedokuto (see page 59)
  Sanoshashinto (see page 70)
  Hochuekkito (see page 61)

ABNORMAL METABOLISM

1. Obesity disorders
2. Diabetes
3. Hyperhidrosis

1. Obesity Disorders

Herbals of choice are

  Bofutsushosanryo
  Daisaikoto (see page 71)

Bofutsushosanryo

A fat person may seem healthy, but he lacks resistance and is frequently in poor physical condition. For a woman, fat detracts from her beauty. The physical characteristics of a fat person are a weak heart and generally high blood pressure; thus it is important to reduce his weight without too much strain. Bofutsushosanryo is effective for the following reactions for a fat person, but it also helps in achieving both health and beauty if a person uses this herb along with careful selection of meals.

Conditions for which the herbal is effective: for a fatty physique with constipation and decrease in the amount of urine, cardiac weakness, arteriosclerosis, high blood pressure, cerebral hemorrhage, habitual constipation, hyperacidity, kidney trouble, and stiff shoulder caused by the previous disorders.

Selection. This herb is effective in removing fat from a person who has a protruding stomach and fat neck, both typical of executives. It is more effective if used in combination with Daisaikoto.

For a person who is bloated with water, appearing either pale or slightly dark and having hyperhidrosis, Boiogito is suggested.

For treatment of overweight, it is important to use herbs, but it is more important to watch meals, avoiding rice, sweet substances or fatty substances, and eating many more vegetables and seaweeds.

2. Diabetes

The herbal of choice is Hachimiganryo (see page 86)

3. Hyperhidrosis

The herbal of choice is Boiogito

Boiogito

Conditions for which the herbal is effective: hyperhidrosis, fatness, arthritis, rheumatism of the joints. For a person who is bloated with water, who looks pale, who tires easily and perspires profusely, or who has edema.

NOTE: This herb is frequently effective for a fat woman of leisure.

ENDOCRINE DISORDERS

Basedow's Disease, Goiter

The herbal of choice is Shakanzoto

Shakanzoto

Conditions for which the herbal is effective: cardiac neurosis, valvular disease of the heart, cough with bloody phlegm, breathing difficulty due to Graves' disease. For a person with bad complexion, anemia, arrhythmia, palpitation, shortness of breath, tendency to constipate, and slight fever.

NOTE: This herb is unsuitable for a person who has a weak stomach with diarrhea.

NERVE, MOTOR NERVE DISORDERS

1. Neuralgia, lumbago
2. Rheumatism, arthritis
3. Stiff shoulders
4. Nervous disorder, neurosis, neurasthenia, insomnia
5. Headache, hot fit, tinnitus aurium
6. Dizziness, vertigo, heavy-headedness

1. Neuralgia, Lumbago

Herbals of choice are

Keishikajutsufuto

Makyoyokukanto
Hachimiganryo (see page 86)

Keishikajutsufuto

Neuralgia and rheumatism are very common conditions in a country like Japan, where the climate is very humid and the difference in temperature between cold and hot is severe. When the metabolism of the body water becomes abnormal due to high humidity in the atmosphere, the unnecessary water content stagnates in the body and lowers the energy-producing metabolic processes; hence a person feels chilly and develops neuralgia or rheumatism. Keishikajutsufuto warms the body, increases metabolism of water content, and is superbly effective for the following reactions.

Conditions for which the herbal is effective: neuralgia, arthritis, and rheumatism. For a person with pain caused by a cold constitution or with ᴊmbness of the hands and legs, or for a person having difficulty in bending and stretching.

Selection. For neuralgia and lumbago: Keishikajutsufuto is effective for general conditions, especially for chronic cases. For a person with acute pain accompanied by chills, the herbalist uses Kakkonto. For a person with severe constipation followed, by cold feet and hips and who has hot fits and develops lumbago, Togakujokito is used. For a person without constipation but having cold hips with pain, Ryokyojutsukanto is used. For a person with severe coldness of the hands and legs with pain in the hips, the herbalist will select either Tokushigyakukagokyoto or Goshakusan. For a person with loss of vitality and having pain in the hips, Hachimiganryo is used. For a person with pain in the joints, Makyoyokukanto is suggested.

For a person with natural perspiration but chilly feeling, either Saikokeishito or Keishito is used. A combination of Deishijutsufuto with Makyoyokukanto is very effective for stubborn cases of neuralgia.

Makyoyokukanto

There are various kinds of rheumatism, such as acute rheumatism of the joints, which swell red and are painful as the climate changes; and rheumatism of the muscle, which is as painful as if the muscle were electrified. Neuralgia also differs according to the location of affliction, such as trigeminal nerve, intercostal nerve, or knucklebone nerve. The causes of rheumatism and neuralgia are not clearly understood, but many people think that they have something important to do with physical characteristics.

Makyoyokukanto is a specialized herb for rheumatism or neuralgia. It has no side effects and removes pain quickly.

Conditions for which the herbal is effective: rheumatism of the joint, rheumatism of the muscle, neuralgia, and warts.

Selection. For rheumatism and arthritis: generally this herb is most widely used in order to effectively remove pain and swelling. For a person with numbness in his hands or feet, the herbalist uses Keishikajutsufuto. For a person with a cold constitution who tires easily, Goshakusan is used. For a person with severe pain, Shakuyakukanzoto may be used for a short period. For a person with swelling who is physically bloated with water, Boiogito is recommended.

Neuralgia: Makyoyokukanto is also used for neuralgia for quick effect (please refer to Keishikajutsufuto, page 000 for further details.)

2. Rheumatism, Arthritis

Herbals of choice are

Makyoyokukanto (see page 94)
Keishikajutsufuto (see page 93)

3. Stiff Shoulders

Herbals of choice are

Kakkonto (see page 47)
Kumibinroto (see page 79)
Daisaikoto (see page 71)
Tokishakuyakusanryo (see page 76)

4. Nervous Disorder, Neurosis, Neurasthenia, Insomnia

Herbals of choice are

Yokukansankachinbihange (see page 80)
Kososan
Saikokaryukotsuboreito (see page 78)
Hangekobokuto (see page 57)

Kososan

Recently the relationship of physical and mental health has been given considerable attention through the study of psycho-physiological medicine. But Oriental herbalism has long known of these effects, as shown by the old saying, "Illness stems from the mind." The mental and nervous reactions are considered especially important and there are many herbals that will control abnormality of the nerves. Kososan is a typical herb that is effective for a person with a relatively weak constitution, for an aged person who has habitual headaches or feels badly, and for persons with a lack of appetite who have neuralgia and colds. It is also effective against urticaria caused by eating shellfish.

Conditions for which the herbal is effective: colds, headache, urticaria, neurasthenia, menopausal neurosis, neural dysmenorrhea. For a person with nervousness, headache, or lack of appetite from feeling badly, and for a person with a heavy-headedness, dizziness, and tinnitus aurium.

Selection. For headache, hot fit, tinnitus aurium: for a person with a lack of appetite due to depression, the herbalist uses Kososan, Saikokaryukotsuboreito, or Keishikaryukotsuboreito. For a person with high blood pressure, Orengedokuto, Kumibinroto, or Sanoshashinto may be used. For a person with physiological disorders, either Keishibukeryoganryo or Togakujokito is used. For a person having a severely dry mouth, Goreisan is used. For a person with fever, Kakkonto, Saikokeishito, or Keishito may be used. For a child with hot fits, Shokenchuto is suggested.

For a person with dizziness from chronic headache, the herbalist uses Reikeijutsukanto. For a person with acute headache, he uses Goshuyuto.

For a person with a cold constitution or anemia, Tokishakuyakusanryo, Tokushigyakukagohoto, or Hochuekkito is recommended.

For a person with dyspepsia, Hangekobokuto or Hangebyakujutsutenmato is used.

5. Headache, Hot Fit, Tinnitus Aurium

Herbals of choice are

Kososan (see page 95)
Kakkonto (see page 47)

Keishibukeryoganryo

Impure blood results when the blood circulation is poor and congestion of blood exists, or when the functioning of the liver to neutralize poisons becomes poor and insufficient removal of waste materials from blood develops. When a female has impure blood, she develops a physiological disorder from irritation of the nerves, including headache, hot fits, and emotional instability, or she develops skin diseases and rough skin texture. Keishibukeryoganryo is effective for reactions throughout the whole body caused by impure blood.

Conditions for which the herbal is effective: Various disorders caused by menozenia, dysmenorrhea, eczema, urticaria, comedones, blemishes, internal bleeding after inflicted by an external wound, bleeding hemorrhoids, impure blood. For a person with hot fits causing congestion of blood in the lower eyelids, headache, tinnitus aurium, stiff shoulders, dizziness, palpitation, chills, and oppressive pain in the lower abdomen.

Selection. For physiological disorders, uterine and ovary conditions, leucorrhea, hot fits: Keishibukeryoganryo is used for a congestive type of person. For a person with constipation, either Togakujokito or Daiobotanpito is appropriate. For a person with heavy leucorrhea, Ryutanshakanto is effective.

For a pale-looking anemic female with female disorders, refer to Tokishakuyakusanryo, page 000.

For bruises and external wounds, the quicker Keishibukeryoganryo is taken, the sooner recovery will occur.

For impure blood: This herb is effective in cleansing

impure blood and is used in combination with other herbals.

6. Dizziness, Vertigo, Heavy-Headedness

Herbals of choice are

Reikeijutsukanto (see page 77)
Kososan (see page 95)
Tokishakuyakusanryo (see page 76)

PEDIATRIC DISORDERS

1. Scrofulosis, underdevelopment.
2. Enuresis or bed-wetting
3. Child asthma
4. Child neurosis, crying at night, fright at night
5. Autointoxication
6. Cervical lymphadenitis, tuberculous adenitis of the hilum

1. Scrofulosis, Underdevelopment

Herbals of choice are

Shosaikoto (see page 52)
Hochuekkito (see page 61)
Shokenchuto (see page 89)

2. Enuresis or Bed-Wetting

Herbals of choice are

Shokenchuto (see page 89)
Hachimiganryo (see page 86)

3. Infantile Asthma

The herbal of choice is

Makyokansekito (see page 56)

4. Infantile Neurosis, Crying at Night, Fright at Night

Herbals of choice are

Shokenchuto (see page 89)
Yokukansankachinbihange (see page 80)

5. Autointoxication

The herbal of choice is Ninjinto

Ninjinto

Conditions for which the herbal is effective: chronic diarrhea, gastritis, gastric atony, anemia, weakness in a child, auto-intoxication, loss of appetite in a child.

For a person with anemia, a cold constitution, oppression of the stomach, stomach pain, tendency to have soft bowel movements or to have diarrhea, often accompanied by heavy-headedness or vomiting.

NOTE: This herbal is used for the purpose of improving the function of the stomach and intestines.

6. Cervical Lymphadenitis, Tuberculous Adenitis of the Hilum

The herbal choice is Sakoseikanto

Conditions for which the herbal is effective: weak constitution, scrofulousness in a child, and also symptoms that accompany these characteristics, such as chronic gastroenteric disorders, anemia, cervical lymphadenitis, tuberculous adenitis of the hilum, enlarged tonsils, nervous disorder, eczema.

NOTE: This herbal is used to improve scrofulousness and is also effective for increasing physical stamina of a weak child who suffers from chronic otitis media.

SURGICAL, DERMATOLOGICAL CONDITIONS

1. Eczema, urticaria, sores
2. Pyosis
3. Comedones
4. Wart
5. Itchy skin
6. Frostbite
7. Blister
8. Bruise, external wounds
9. Keratosis of the palm
10. Loss of hair

1. Eczema, Urticaria, Sores

Herbals of choice are

Jumiheidokuto
Keishibukeryoganryo (see page 97)
Seijobofuto

Jumiheidokuto

In the field of medicine, one of the things Japan can be proud of is that it had a doctor of Oriental herbalism, Seishu Hamaoka, who was the first to use a general anesthetic in performing a major operation. Jumiheidokuto is a modern herbal developed from the traditional herbal called Jumiheidokuto, which was originated by Dr. Seishu Hamaoka for internal use for skin diseases. This herbal is very effective for improvement of physical conditions that underlie skin diseases, stimulates immunological functions and drainage of pus, and acts internally.

Conditions for which the herbal is effective: pus-containing swellings, eczema, urticaria, comedones, improvement of physical characteristics in furunculosis (tendency to develop pus-containing sores).

Selection. For eczema, urticaria, pus-containing sores: this herbal is effective except at the beginning. For a person with a physiological disorder (vague symptoms), a combination of this herb with Keishibukeryoganryo is used. For a woman who wants to beautify her skin texture, a combination of this herb with Yokuininkotaro* is suggested. For a person with urticaria caused by food poisoning, Inchinkoto or Kososan is used. For a person with hypersecretion, Eppikajutsuto is used. For a person with early reactions of feverishness, the herbalist uses Kakkonto. For a person having facial eczema with comedones, he will use Seijobofuto. For a person with impure blood accompanied by constipation, the herbalist uses either Togakujokito or Daiobotanpito. For an aged person or a person with diabetes and eczema, he uses Hachimiganryo. For infantile neurosis with eczema, he uses Saikoseikanto. For a person with genital eczema, Ryutanshakanto is recommended. For a person with a stubborn skin condition, a combination of Jumiheidokuto and either Shofusan or Hainosankyuto is effective.

Comedones (blackheads) are the enemy of beauty and source of worry for young men and women. They are caused by maladjustment of sexual hormones, gastroenteric disorders, constipation, etc. Seijobofuto, a new Oriental herbal in tablet form, works on the internal disorders that cause comedones. It is made from the combined essence of eleven herbs that are effective in strengthening the stomach, the intestines and the liver, in promoting antitoxins, and in adjusting bowel movement. It stops hypersecretion of smegma, heals inflammation. removes pus, and in a short time cures such unpleasant disorders as comedones, facial eczema, and facial furuncles (skin eruptions).

Conditions for which the herbal is effective: comedones, facial eczema.

Selection. This herb is effective in general for both men and women. However, for a person with a physiological disorder, Keishibukeryoganryo or a combination of Keishibukeryoganryo and Seijobofuto is recommended. For a person with a physiological disorder accompanied by constipation, the herbalist will choose either Togakujokito or Daiobotanpito or a combination of one of these herbals with Seijobofuto. For an anemic middle-aged woman with a cold constitution who is bothered by comedones, Tokishakuyakusanryo or a combination of Tokishakuyakusanryo and Seijobofuto is recommended. For comedones and eczema that are incurable by these herbs, Jumiheidokuto in many instances has worked effectively, and also a combination of Jumiheidokuto and Yokuinin is used.

2. Pyosis

Herbals of choice are

Kikyosekko
Hainosankyuto

Kikyosekko

This herb is an additive used to enforce the removal of inflammation, pus, and phlegm from various inflammations, such as otitis media or tonsillitis.

Conditions for which the herbal is effective: removal of phlegm, discharge of pus.

Hainosankyuto

Conditions for which the herbal is effective: pyosis accompanied by red blotches and swelling of the affected area, boils, carbuncles on the face, and other sores.

NOTE: This herb is used while the suppurative swelling is painful and the affected area is still hard.

3. Comedones

Herbals of choice are

Seijobofuto (see page 102)
Keishibukeryoganryo (see page 97)
Jumiheidokuto (see page 100)

4. Warts

Herbals of choice are

Makyoyokukanto (see page 94)
Yokuinin

This herb is famous because it is used internally for the removal of warts; it cures skin conditions and is effective in building a beautiful skin complexion when combined with other herbs.

Conditions for which the herbal is effective: abnormal urination, removal of inflammation, tranquilizer for the removal of warts. Effective for skin conditions.

5. Itchy Skin

Herbals of choice are

Orengedokuto (see page 59)
Shishihakuhito

Shishihakuhito

Conditions for which the herbal is effective: jaundice, pruritis, hangover. For a person with oppression of the liver.

NOTE: Laxating a person with a damaged liver is contraindicated.

6. Frostbite

Herbals of choice are

Tokushigyakukagokyoto
Tokishakuyakusanryo (see page 76)

Tokushigyakukagokyoto

The first stage of frostbite is that the affected portion becomes red and itches; the second stage is that it breaks open and becomes festered; the third stage is that it becomes rotten and black and sometimes develops into an ulcer. Frostbite occurs when heat is removed from the skin in cold temperatures, and new blood cannot reach the periphery of the fingers or toes because of poor circulation. Tokushigyakukagokyoto is an herb that increases the circulation of the blood, warms the body, and promotes blood circulation to the periphery of the body. It not only treats and prevents frostbite, but also is effective for the following conditions.

Conditions for which the herbal is effective: frostbite, chronic headache, sciatica, female abdominal pain. For a person with anemia, a cold constitution accompanied by headache, heavy oppressive feeling in the stomach. For a person with lumbago or abdominal pain who suffers easily from frostbite.

Selection. This herb is noted for the treatment and prevention of frostbite, and helps quick recovery from soreness and gangrene. This herbal should be taken regularly beginning in autumn for preventive care. Tokishakuyakusanryo may be used in addition.

7. Blister

The herbal of choice is Eppikajutso (see page 83)

8. Bruise, External Wound

The herbal of choice is Keishibukeryoganryo (see page 97)

9. Keratosis of the Palm

The herbal of choice is Tokushigyakukagokyoto (see page 104)

10. Loss of Hair

The herbal of choice is Saikokaryukotsuboreito (see page 78)

ANAL CONDITIONS

Piles, Proctocele, Bleeding of Hemorrhoids

Herbals of choice are

Otsujito
Tokishakuyakusanryo (see page 76)
Hochuekkito (see page 61)

Otsujito

The causes of piles are habitual constipation, pregnancy, and the Japanese style of sitting, all of which contribute to the interruption of blood circulation. Also, a tendency to develop piles may be inherited. Almost all of the medicines for external application are temporary deterrents, and do not cure completely the root cause; therefore, it is necessary to take herbals for internal use, which act effectively in these complex causes.

Otsujito is a herbal modernized from the traditional Oriental herbal also called Otsujito. It is intended for internal use with piles and proctocele and removes quickly troubles caused by pain or bleeding.

Conditions for which the herbal is effective: hemorrhoids, proctocele, bleeding of the anus, excruciating pain from piles.

Selection. This herb stops the pain and bleeding of piles and is specially prepared for internal use for fast results. It is *not* suitable for a person who is usually bothered by diarrhea. For such a person choose Tokishakuyakusanryo or Hochuekkito, depending on his physical characteristics.

For a person with anemia caused by loss of blood from bleeding of piles, Kyukikyogaito and Hochuekkito are more effective. A combination of Otsujito with an herb for external application will not cause any ill effects.

GYNECOLOGICAL DISORDERS

1. Vague complaints, disorders of the female reproductive organs, leucorrhea, conditions related to childbirth
2. Menopause, female dizziness
3. Morning sickness
4. Cold constitution
5. Mastitis
6. Vaginitis, pudendal eczema, pruritus
7. Impure blood

1. Vague Complaints, Disorders of the Female Reproductive Organs, Leucorrhea, Conditions Related to Childbirth

Herbals of choice are

Keishibukeryoganryo (see page 97)
Tokishakuyakusanryo (see page 76)
Togakujokito
Shimotsuto

Togakujokito

In Oriental herbalism, the cause of illness is categorized in the following three general classifications: (1) "Ki," (2) "Ketsu" or "Chi," and (3) "Sui" or "Misu."

"Ki" means feeling and represents blood circulation; "Ketsu" or "Chi" means vital fluid. "Misu" means water and represents metabolism of water content.

The following list of conditions for which the herbal is effective are mostly caused by "Chi" effects. Togakujokito is effective for especially severe reactions caused by the "Chi" disorders and is used for a person with a strong physique who has constipation.

Conditions for which the herbal is effective: various kinds of disorders due to menoxenia, menopausal disorders, leucorrhea, hemorrhoids, comedones, blemishes, eczema, lumbago, sciatica, high blood pressure, arteriosclerosis, habitual constipation. For a person tending to have headaches or hot fits, with oppressive pain at the lower left side of the abdomen or constipation, with cold lower limbs or hips and whose amount of urination decreases.

Selection. For menopausal disorders and female dizziness, Togakujokito is effective for a person with a reddish dark face who has constipation.

For a person with anemia who has a cold constitution, either Tokishakuyakusanryo or Shimotsuto is suggested.

For a person with lumbago who urinates a large amount and complains of thirst, Hachimiganryo is recommended.

For a person with severe nervousness which causes constriction of the chest and throat, Hangekobokuto is used.

For a person with insomnia having constipation, Saikokaryukotsuboreito or Kamishoyosan is used.

For a person with debility, Saikokeishikankyoto is effective. For a person with high blood pressure who is emotionally unstable, Yokukansankachinbihange is suggested. For a woman with various unstable disorders

108

during menopause, Saikokeishito is effective in many cases.

Shimotsuto

Conditions for which the herbal is effective: anemia, menopausal disorder, menoxenia, menostasis, menorrhagia, conditions related to childbirth, high blood pressure. For a person with anemia, a cold constitution, a weak but rather stuffy stomach, and a tendency to constipate.

NOTE: This herb improves blood circulation, treats anemia, and is a basic herb frequently combined with others.

2. Menopause, Female Dizziness

Herbals of choice are

Saikokeishito (see page 50)
Togakujokito (see page 107)
Tokishakuyakusanryo (see page 76)
Yokukansankachinbihange (see page 80)

3. Morning Sickness

Herbals of choice are

Hangekobokuto (see page 57)
Hangeshashinto (see page 66)

4. Cold Constitution

Herbals of choice are

Tokishakuyakusanryo (see page 76)

Keishibukeryoganryo (see page 97)
Tokushigyakukagokyoto (see page 104)
Hachimiganryo (see page 86)

5. Mastitis

The herbal of choice is Kakkonto (see page 47)

6. Vaginitis, Pudendal Eczema, Pruritus

The herbal of choice is Ryutanshakanto

Ryutanshakanto

Conditions for which the herbal is effective: for a person with some physical stamina and who has the following reactions: urethritis, catarrh of the bladder, vaginitis, genital eczema, leucorrhea, genital itchiness, and endometritis.

NOTE: For a person especially with debility, use Tokishakuyakusanryo.

7. Impure Blood

The herbal of choice is Keishibukeryoganryo (see page 97)

OTORHINOLARYNGOLOGICAL CONDITIONS

1. Ozena, rhinitis, clogging of the nose
2. Tympanitis
3. Tonsillitis

1. Ozena, Rhinitis, Clogging of the Nose

Herbals of choice are

110

Kakkontakashinisenkyu (see page 49)
Noza C

Noza C

The cavities that connect with the main nasal cavity are called the sinus cavities. When pus accumulates in the accessory cavities of a person with allergy, it is called empyema. Of these cavities, it is easy to remove pus from the upper jaw cavity and from the ethmoid cavity, but it is difficult to operate on the frontal cavity, which spreads from the center of the eyebrows to the forehead, or on the butterfly-shaped cavity in the skull in the back of the nasal cavity. Noza C is an Oriental herbal for internal use in difficult-to-treat cases of ozena and is very effective when continuously used over a long period: it is very effective against such unpleasant reactions as headache, loss of memory, and feeling of fatigue due to ozena.

Conditions for which the herbal is effective: ozena, chronic rhinitis, clogging of the nose.

Selection. For ozena and clogging of the nose: generally ozena becomes chronic, and Noza C is prepared especially for chronic and difficult cases. There are many instances where Kakkontokashinisenkyu is better suited than Noza C for normal ozena. For a person with thick nasal mucus, a combination of Noza C with Kikyosekko is used.

For further difficult reactions, a combination of Noza C with Hakushusan (consisting of viper, tsu-crab, and rhinoceros horn charred together) is effective sometimes. Please refer to the "Selection" section of Kakkonto, page 48, for other usages.

111

2. Tympanitis

The herbal of choice is Saikoseikanto (see page 100)

3. Tonsillitis

The herbal of choice is Kakkonto (see page 47)

OPHTHALMOLOGICAL CONDITIONS

Conjunctivitis, Lacryoadenitis

Herbals of choice are

Kakkonto (see page 47)
Shoseiryuto (see page 53)

OTHER DISORDERS

1. Adynamia, debility, loss of weight, anemia, night sweating
2. Fatigue and weariness
3. Constitutional improvement

1. Adynamia, Debility, Loss of Weight, Anemia, Night Sweating

Herbals of choice are

Juzentaihoto (see page 81)
Shosaikoto (see page 52)

2. Fatigue and Weariness

Herbals of choice are

Kumibinroto (see page 79)
Daisaikoto (see page 71)

Hachimiganryo (see page 86)
Hochuekkito (see page 61)

3. Constitutional Improvement

Herbals of choice are

Shosaikoto (see page 52)
Daisaikoto (see page 71)

OTHER ORIENTAL HERBAL COMPOSITIONS

Bukuryoin

Conditions for which the herbal is effective: dilation of the stomach, sore stomach, gastritis, gastric atony, gastric nervous disorder, indigestion. For a person with a constricted stuffy feeling in the stomach, excessive secretion of gastric juice, nausea, vomiting, loss of appetite, and small amount of urine.

NOTE: This herb is used for diarrhea or conversely for constipation with the above conditions.

Byokukokaninjinto

Conditions for which the herbal is effective: habitual constipation, acute constipation, high blood pressure, food-poisoning. For a person who feels severe constriction in the abdomen, who is constipated, or who is fat and constipated.

NOTE: This herb is used especially for stubborn constipation but is unsuitable for a weak person.

Daisaikotokyodaio

Conditions for which the herbal is effective: gastroenteric disorders, bronchial asthma, jaundice, cholelithiasis, cholecystitis, high blood pressure, arteriosclerosis, hemiplegia, insomnia, impotence, pleurisy, neurasthenia. For a person who feels tense in the pit of the stomach; feels pain or oppression in the chest, at the side of the abdomen, or in the liver; suffers from tinitus aurium, stiff shoulders, or fatigue, often with loss of appetite; or has constipation.

NOTE: This herb differs from Daisaikoto in that the laxative, Daio, has been extracted.

Dokudami

Conditions for which the herbal is effective: neutralizing toxins, constipation, for urination during urethritis, decrease in the amount of urination, pain during urination, swelling of the hips and legs, nephritis.

NOTE: This herbal is famous as an antitoxic substance. It may be used alone or in combination with other herbs.

Goshakusan

Conditions for which the herbal is effective: This herbal is used for the following main reactions in persons with a cold constitution, a tendency to be easily fatigued, and a weak stomach and intestines: lumbago, sciatica, rheumatism, beriberi, gynecological disorders, gastritis, gastric atony, dilatation of the stomach.

NOTE: This herb is effective for above reactions caused by cold weather or moist humidity.

Hangebyakujutsutenmato

Conditions for which the herbal is effective: gastric atony, headache stemming from a weak stomach and intestines or from low blood pressure, dizziness. For a person with a cold constitution or atonic constitution who tires easily, and who has headache, heavy-headedness, dizziness, and stiff shoulders, accompanied by chills or vomiting.

Kamishoyosan

Conditions for which the herbal is effective: nervous disorders, insomnia, menopausal disorders, menoxenia, nervousness of the stomach, gastric atony, dilatation of the stomach, constipation, eczema. For a person with headache, heavy-headedness, hot fits, stiff shoulders, feeling of constant fatigue, loss of appetite, and constipation.

NOTE: This herb is especially effective for those who have hot fits and a flushed face.

Kanbakutaisoto

Conditions for which the herbal is effective: neurasthenia, palpitation, sexual neurosis, impotence, child's bed-wetting, night fright, alopecia. For a person with nervous disorders, headache, hot fits, tinnitus aurium, who is easily fatigued and notices throbbing around the hips, and who has increased frequency of urination as well as increased amount of urine.

NOTE: This herb is very suitable for the above reactions in youths or old persons.

Keishito

Conditions for which the herbal is effective: colds, headache, neuralgia, rheumatism of the joints or the muscles, neurasthenia. For a person with natural perspiration and a slight fever or chills.

NOTE: This herbal is a basic ingredient in other Oriental herbals, and is often used in combination with other herbs.

Kyukikyogaito

Conditions for which the herbal is effective: bleeding hemorrhoids, internal bleeding from external wounds, bleeding after childbirth, anemia. For a person with a cold constitution and anemia caused by excessive bleeding.

NOTE: For a person with extreme debility, use Juzentaihoto.

Maosaishinbushito

Conditions for which the herbal is effective: cold, cough, asthma. For a person with frequent phlegm, chills, and breathing difficulty.

NOTE: This herb is effective for the above reactions in an aged or weak person.

Mokuboito

Conditions for which the herbal is effective: endocarditis, valvular disease of the heart, cardiac asthma, chronic nephritis, nephrosis. For a person who feels a constriction in the pit of the stomach, who has difficult breathing and stridor, who has edema with a small amount of urine, and who is dry in the mouth or throat.

NOTE: This herb seems to be more effective for people who have a pale-dark facial texture.

Ninjinyoeito

Conditions for which the herbal is effective: improvement of physical stamina in a weak body, treatment after illness or after childbirth. For a person with thin physique, poor complexion, slight fever, chills, persistent cough, continuous fatigue, loss of appetite, emotional instability, insomnia, night sweating, and a tendency to constipate.

NOTE: This herb is effective for serious conditions such as tuberculosis, which causes debility and shows the above reactions.

Orento

Conditions for which the herbal is effective: catarrh of the stomach and intestines, stomatitis, indigestion, hyperacidity, hangover. For a person with oppression of the stomach, loss of appetite, abdominal pain, nausea, vomiting, bad breath and coated tongue, constipation, or diarrhea.

NOTE: This herb is effective for acute and severe reactions. For constipation, a combination of Orento with Daio (Rheum) is used.

Ryokankyomishingeninto

Conditions for which the herbal is effective: bronchitis, bronchial asthma, cardiac weakness, kidney trouble.

117

For a person with anemia, a cold constitution, and cough with stridor and much phlegm.

NOTE: This herb is used by a person with the above reactions who cannot take any herb that includes Maoto.

Ryokyojutsukanto

Conditions for which the herbal is effective: sciatica, lumbago, cold hips, bed-wetting. For a person with a feeling of weary fatigue all over the body, pain and chills and a heavy feeling in the hips with increasing frequency of urination as well as increases in amount of urine.

NOTE: This herb is used for a person with coldness of the feet and hips that feels as though he were sitting in water.

Saikanto

Conditions for which the herbal is effective: bronchitis, chest pain caused by pleurisy, bronchial asthma. For a person with chest pain, back pain, hydrothorax, constriction in the chest or in the stomach or decrease in the amount of urination, or for a person who coughs out sticky sputum.

NOTE: This herb is used for the purpose of removing chest pain or hydrothorax.

Shakuyakukanzoto*

Conditions for which the herbal is effective: tension of the rectus abdominis; stomachache or abdominal pain; spastic pain due to cholelithiasis, nephrolithiasis, or cystolith; muscle and joint pains of the limbs; abdominal pain due to the side effect of medication; gastric cramp; acute stomach pain.

Shinbuto

Conditions for which the herbal is effective: catarrh of the colon. For a person with diarrhea, abdominal pain, nausea, slight bowel movement, palpitation, or very cold hands and feet.

NOTE: This herb is suitable for a physically weak person who lacks vitality.

Shishihakuhito

Conditions for which the herbal is effective: jaundice, pruritus, hangover. For a person with oppression of the liver.

NOTE: This herb is suitable for the above conditions, for which a laxative is unsuitable.

Shofusan

Conditions for which the herbal is effective: stubborn skin condition over a period of years. If the affected area is dry or has a thin secretion, or if the area easily changes during summer or during a warm period.

NOTE: This herb is frequently effective for stubborn skin conditions that other herbs have failed to relieve.

Shohangekabukuryoto

Conditions for which the herbal is effective: morning sickness, vomiting. For a person who feels stagnation of water in the stomach and vomits.

NOTE: This herb is taken a little at a time and frequently.

APPENDIX A:
Partial List of Herbal Compositions

(1) ANCHUSANRYO	grams		grams
		Zingiber	3
Cinnamomum	4	Glycyrrhiza	1.5
Corydalis	3		
Ostrea testa	3	(5) BUKURYOIN	
Foeniculum	1.5	Hoelen	5
Glycyrrhiza	1	Panax	3
Alpinia	0.5	Atractylodes	4
		Aurantium	1.5
		Citrus	3
(2) BAKUMONTO		Zingiber	3
Ophiopogon	10		
Pinella	5	(6) BYOKUKOKANINJINTO	
Panax	2	Gypsum	15
Zizyphus	3	Anemarrhena	5
Glycyrrhiza	2	Oryza	8
Oryza	5	Glycyrrhiza	2
		Panax	1.5
(3) BOFUTSUSHOSANRYO			
Ligusticum	1.2	(7) CHOREITO	
Paeonia	1.2	Polyporus	3
Gardenia	1.2	Hoelen	3
Cunidium	1.2	Alisma	3
Porstythia	1.2	Glutin	3
Nepeta	1.2	Talcum	3
Ephedra	1.2		
Glehnia	1.2		
Zingiber	1.2	(8) CHOYOTO	
Rheum	1.5	Coix	9
Mentha	1.2	Benincasa	6
Platycodon	2	Persica	5
Scutellaria	2	Moutan	4
Glycyrrhiza	2		
Talcum	3	(9) DAIJOKITO	
Gypsum	2	Rheum	2
Magnesia	1.5	Magnolia	5
		Aurantium	3
		Magnesia	3
(4) BOIOGITO			
Astragalus	5		
Atractylodes	3	(10) DAIKENCHUTO	
Zizyphus	3	Zanthoxylum	2

	grams		grams
Zingiber	5	Hoelen	4.5
Panax	3	Atractylodes	4.5
Dulcium	20	Alisma	6
		Cinnamomum	3

(18) GOSHAKUSAN

Rheum	2	**(11) DAIO**	
		Ligusticum	2
(12) DAIOBOTANPITO		Cunidium	1
Rheum	2	Paeonia	1
Moutan	4	Atractylodes	2
Persica	4	Magnolia	1
Benincasa	6	Citrus	2
Magnesia	4	Hoelen	2
		Angelica	1
(13) DAISAIKOTO		Aurantium	1
Bupleurum	6	Platycodon	1
Scutellaria	3	Zingiber	1
Pinella	4	Pinella	2
Paeonia	3	Cinnomomum	1
Aurantium	2	Ephedra	1
Zingiber	4	Zizyphus	1
Zizyphus	3	Glycyrrhiza	1
Rheum	1 or 2		

(14) DAISAIKOTOKYODAIO		**(19) GOSHUYUTO**	
		Evodia	3
Bupleurum	6	Ginseng	2
Scutellaria	3	Zizyphus	4
Pinella	4	Zingiber	4
Paeonia	3		
Aurantium	2	**(20) HACHIMIGANRYO**	
Zingiber	4	Rehmannia	5
Zizyphus	3	Dioscorea	3
		Cornus	3
(15) DOKUDAMI		Alisma	3
		Hoelen	3
(16) EPPIKAJUTSUTO		Moutan	3
Ephedra	6	Cinnamomum	1
Zingiber	3		
Glycyrrhiza	4		
Gypsum	8	**(21) HAINOSANKYUTO**	
Zizyphus	3	Aurantium	3
		Platycodon	3
(17) GOREISAN		Paeonia	3
Polyporus	4.5	Zingiber	3

	grams
Zizyphus	6
Glycyrrhiza	3

(22) HANGEBYAKUJUTSU-TENMATO

	grams
Pinella	3
Citrus	3
Hordeum	2
Hoelen	3
Astragalus	1.5
Panax	1.5
Alisma	1.5
Gastrodia	2
Atractylodes	3
Gnaphalium	2
Phellandrium	1
Zingiber	2

(23) HANGEKOBOKUTO

	grams
Pinella	6
Hoelen	5
Magnolia	3
Perilla	2
Zingiber	4

(24) HANGESHASHINTO

	grams
Pinella	5
Scutellaria	2.5
Panax	2.5
Zizyphus	2.5
Zingiber	2.5
Glycyrrhiza	2.5

(25) HEISANRYO

	grams
Atractylodes	4
Magnolia	3
Citrus	3
Zizyphus	2
Zingiber	2
Glycyrrhiza	1

(26) HOCHUEKKITO

	grams
Astragalus	3
Panax	3
Atractylodes	3
Ligusticum	3
Citrus	2
Zingiber	2
Zizyphus	2
Bupleurum	2
Cimicifuga	1
Glycyrrhiza	1.5

(27) INCHINKOTO

	grams
Artemisia	4
Gardenia	3
Rheum	1

(28) JUMIHEIDOKUTO

	grams
Bupleurum	2
Platycodon	2
Phelloptorus	1.5
Cunidium	2
Prunus	2
Scutellaria	2
Zingiber	2
Angelica	1.5

(29) JUZENTAIHOTO

	grams
Panax	2.5
Atractylodes	3.5
Hoelen	3.5
Glycyrrhiza	1
Rehmannia	3.5
Paeonia	3
Ligusticum	3.5
Cunidium	3
Cinnamomum	3
Astragalus	2.5

(30) KAKKONTO

	grams
Pueraria	8
Ephedra	4
Zingiber	4
Cinnamomum	3
Paeonia	3
Glycyrrhiza	4
Zizyphus	2

(31) KAKKONTOKASHINIS-ENKYU

Pueraria	8
Ephedra	4
Zingiber	4
Cinnamomum	3
Paeonia	3
Glycyrrhiza	2
Zizyphus	4
Cunidium	3
Magnolia	3

(32) KAMISHOYOSAN

Ligusticum	3
Paeonia	3
Bupleurum	3
Atractylodes	3
Hoelen	3
Zingiber	2
Glycyrrhiza	1.5
Mentha	1
Moutan	2
Gardenia	2

(33) KANBAKUTAISOTO

Glycyrrhiza	5
Zizyphus	6
Fructus	20

(34) KEISHIBUKERYO-GANRYO

Cinnamomum	4
Hoelen	4
Moutan	4
Persica	4
Paeonia	4

(35) KEISHIKAJUTSUFUTO

Paeonia	4
Zizyphus	4
Zingiber	4
Glycyrrhiza	2
Atractylodes	5

(36) KEISHIKARYUKOTSU-BOREITO

Paeonia	4
Zingiber	4
Glycyrrhiza	2
Zizyphus	4
Os stegodontis	3
Ostrea testa	3

(37) KEISHIKASHAKUYA-KUTO

Cinnamomum	4
Paeonia	6
Zingiber	4
Glycyrrhiza	2
Zizyphus	4

(38) KEISHITO

Cinnamomum	4
Paeonia	4
Zizyphus	4
Zingiber	4
Glycyrrhiza	2

(39) KIKYOSEKKO

Platycodon	1
Gypsum	1

(40) KOSOSAN

Perilla	1
Cyperus	4
Citrus	2.5
Glycyrrhiza	1
Zingiber	3

(41) KUMIBINROTO

Areca	4
Magnolia	3
Cinnamomum	3
Citrus	3
Costi	1
Glycyrrhiza	1
Perilla	1.5

	grams		grams

	grams
Evodia	1
Hoelen	3
(42) KYUKIKYOGAITO	
Ligusticum	4.5
Cinidium	3
Paeonia	4.5
Rehmannia	6
Glutin	3
Artemisia	3
Glycyrrhiza	3
(43) MAKYOKANSEKITO	
Ephedra	4
Armeniaca	4
Glycyrrhiza	2
Gypsum	10
(44) MAKYOYOKUKANTO	
Ephedra	3
Armeniaca	3
Coix	10
Glycyrrhiza	2
(45) MAOSAISHINBUSHITO	
Ephedra	4
Asarum	3
(46) MAOTO	
Ephedra	5
Cinnamomum	4
Armeniaca	5
Glycyrrhiza	1.5
(47) MASHININGANRYO	
Rheum	4
Paeonia	2
Aurantium	2
Magnolia	2
Armeniaca	2
(48) MOKUBOITO	
Gypsum	10
Cinnamomum	3
Panax	3

	grams
(49) NINJINTO	
Panax	3
Atractylodes	3
Zingiber	3
Glycyrrhiza	3
(50) NINJINYOEITO	
Bupleurum	6
Hoelen	4
Platycodon	3
Panax	3
Fritillaria	2
Clutinum	3
Armeniaca	2
Morus	3
Citrus	1.5
Schizandra	1.5
Glycyrrhiza	1.5
(51) NOZA C	
Ephedra	8
Pueraria	4
Cinnamomum	3
Zingiber	4
Fructus	2
Zizyphus	4
Paeonia	3
Magnolia	3
Cunidium	3
(52) ORENGEDOKUTO	
Coptis	3
Phellandrium	2
Scutellaria	2
Gardenia	1
(53) ORENTO	
Coptis	3
Glycyrrhiza	3
Zingiber	3
Panax	3
Cinnamomum	3
Zizyphus	3
Pinella	6

(54) OTSUJITO

Bupleurum	5
Ligusticum	6
Scutellaria	3
Cimicifuga	1.5
Rheum	1
Glycyrrhiza	2

(55) REIKEIJUTSUKANTO

Hoelen	6
Cinnamomum	4
Atractylodes	3
Glycyrrhiza	2

(56) RIKKUNSHITO

Panax	4
Atractylodes	4
Hoelen	4
Glycyrrhiza	1
Pinella	4
Citrus	2
Zingiber	2
Zizyphus	2

(57) RYOKANKYOMISH-INGENINTO

Hoelen	4
Glycyrrhiza	2
Zingiber	2
Schizandra	3
Asarum	2
Pinella	4
Armeniaca	4

(58) RYOKYOJUTSUKANTO

Hoelen	6
Zingiber	3
Atractylodes	3

(59) RYUTANSHAKANTO

Ligusticum	5
Rehmannia	5
Scutellaria	3
Gardenia	1.5
Plantago	3
Alisma	3
Glycyrrhiza	1.5
Akeba	5

(60) SAIKANTO

Bupleurum	5
Pinella	5
Scutellaria	3
Zingiber	3
Zizyphus	3
Trichosanthis	3
Glycyrrhiza	1.5
Coptis	1.5
Panax	2

(61) SAIKOKARYUKOTSU-BOREITO

Bupleurum	5
Pinella	4
Scutellaria	2.5
Cinnamomum	3
Hoelen	3
Os stegondontis	2.5
Ostrea testa	2.5
Zizyphus	2.5
Zingiber	2.5
Ginseng	2.5
Rheum	1

(62) SAIKOKEISHIKAN-KYOTO

Bupleurum	6
Cinnamomum	3
Scutellaria	3
Trichosanthis	3
Ostrea testa	3
Zingiber	2
Glycyrrhiza	2

(63) SAIKOKEISHITO

Bupleurum	5
Scutellaria	2

	grams		grams
Pinella	4	Zingiber	3
Panax	2	Cinnamomum	3
Cinnamomum	2.5	Ophiopogon	6
Paeonia	2	Rehmannia	6
Zingiber	2	Zizyphus	3
Glycyrrhiza	1.5	Panax	3
Zizyphus	2	Glutin	2

(64) SAIKOSEIKANTO

Ligusticum	1.5
Paeonia	1.5
Cunidium	1.5
Rehmannia	1.5
Forsythia	1.5
Platycodon	1.5
Arctium	1.5
Trichosanthis	1.5
Mentha	1.5
Glycyrrhiza	1.5
Phellandrium	1.5
Scutellaria	1.5
Gardenia	1.5
Bupleurum	2

(65) SANOSHASHINTO

Rheum	1
Coptis	1
Scutellaria	1

(66) SEIJOBOFUTO

Glehnia	2.5
Nepeta	1
Forsythia	2.5
Gardenia	2
Coptis	1
Scutellaria	2.5
Citrus	1.5
Angelica	2.5
Platycodon	2.5
Glycyrrhiza	1.5
Mentha	1

(67) SHAKANZOTO

Glycyrrhiza	3

(68) SHIMOTSUTO

Ligusticum	3
Cunidium	3
Paeonia	3
Rehmannia	3

(69) SHINBUTO

Hoelen	5
Paeonia	3
Atractylodes	3
Zingiber	3

(70) SHINPITO

Ephedra	5
Perilla	1.5
Citrus	2.5
Bupleurum	2
Armeniaca	4
Magnolia	3
Glycyrrhiza	2

(71) SHISHIHAKUHITO

Gardenia	3
Glycyrrhiza	1
Phellandrium	2

(72) SHOFUSAN

Ligusticum	3
Rehmannia	3
Gypsum	3
Glehnia	2
Atractylodes	2
Akebia	2
Arctium	2
Cicoda shell	1
Anemarrhena	1.5

Sesamum	1.5
Nepeta	1
Sophora	1
Glycyrrhiza	1

(73) SHOHANGEKABUKURY-OTO

Pinella	6
Zingiber	6
Hoelen	5

(74) SHOKENCHUTO

Cinnamomum	4
Paeonia	6
Zizyphus	4
Zingiber	4
Glycyrrhiza	2
Dulcium	20

(75) SHOSAIKOTO

Bupleurum	7
Pinella	5
Scutellaria	3
Ginseng	3
Zizyphus	3
Zingiber	4
Glycyrrhiza	2

(76) SHOSEIRYUTO

Ephedra	3
Paeonia	3
Asarum	3
Zingiber	3
Glycyrrhiza	3
Cinnamomum	3
Schizandra	3
Pinella	6

(77) TOGAKUJOKITO

Persica	5
Cinnamomum	4
Rheum	3
Magnesia	2
Glycyrrhiza	1.5

(78) TOKISHAKUYAKU-SANRYO

Ligusticum	3
Paeonia	4
Cunidium	3
Atractylodes	4
Hoelen	4
Alisma	4

(79) TOKUSHIGYAKUKAGO-KYOTO

Ligusticum	3
Cinnamomum	3
Paeonia	3
Asarum	2
Glycyrrhiza	2
Akebia	3
Zizyphus	5
Evodia	2
Zinziber	5

(80) YOKUKANSANKACH-INBIHANGE

Ligusticum	3
Atractylodes	4
Hoelen	4
Uncaria	3
Cunidum	3
Bupleurum	2
Glycyrrhizae	2
Pinella	5
Citrus	3

APPENDIX B:
Herbs and Their Properties

The following herbs are well known in Western countries.

Herb	Latin Name	English Common Name	Plant Part Used	Medicinal Property
alisma	Alisma plantago	water plantain	leaves	diuretic, diaphoretic
alpinia	Alpinia officianarum	galangal	rhizome	carminative, stimulant
angelica	Angelica archangelica	garden angelica	root, seeds, herb	aromatic stimulant
arctium	Arctium lappa	burdock	root, herb, seeds (fruits)	alterative, diuretic
areca	Areca catechu	areca nut	seed	astringent, taenicide
artemisia	Artemisia absinthium	wormwood	herb	tonic, stomachic
asarum	Asarum canadense	wild ginger	rhizome	expectorant carminative
astragalus	Astragalus gummifer	tragacanth	gummy exudation	mucilaginous, demulcent

Herb	Latin Name	English Common Name	Plant Part Used	Medicinal Property
aurantium	Citrus aurantium	bitter orange	fruit rind, oil, flowers	tonic, stomachic
cimicifuga	Cimicifuga racemosa	black cohosh	rhizome	astringent, alterative
cinnamomum	Cinnamomum zeylanicum	cinnamon	bark	carminative, astringent
citrus	Citrus reticulata			
coix		Job's tears		
coptis	Coptis trifolia	gold thread	rhizome	bitter tonic
cornus	Cornus mas	cornelian cherry		
corydalis	Dicentra canadensis	turkey corn	root	diuretic, alterative
cyperus	Cyperus articulatus	adrue	root	sedative antiemetic
dioscorea	Dioscorea villosa	wild yam	root	antibilious antispasmodic

130

Herb	Latin Name	English Common Name	Plant Part Used	Medicinal Property
ephedra	Ephedra sinica	ephedra	stem	relief of asthma and hay fever
foeniculum	Foeniculum vulgare	fennel	fruit	stimulant, carminative
gardenia	Gardenia florida			
glycyrrhiza	Glycyrrhiza glabra	licorice, laquiritia	root	pectoral, emollient
gnaphalium	Gnaphalium uliginosum	cudweed	herb	astringent
hordeum	Hordeum vulgare	barley	decorticated seeds	nutritive, demulcent
inula	Inula helenium	elecampane	root	diuretic, expectorant
ligusticum	Ligusticum levisticum	lovage	root	diuretic, carminative
magnolia	Magnolia virginiana	magnolia	bark	stimulant, tonic
mentha	Mentha piperita	peppermint	herb	stimulant, carminative

131

Herb	Latin Name	English Common Name	Plant Part Used	Medicinal Property
morus	Morus nigra	mulberry	fruit	nutritive, refrigerant
nepeta	Nepeta cataria	catnip	herb	carminative, tonic
ophiopogon	Ophioglossum vulgatum	adder's tongue	herb	antiscrofulous, emollient
oryza	Oryza sativa	rice	seeds	nutritive, demulcent
panax	Panax quinquefolium	ginseng	root	tonic, stimulant
paeonia	Paeonia officinalis	peony	root	antispasmodic, tonic
pareira (pueraria)	Chondodendron tomentosum	pareira	root	tonic, diuretic
persica	Prunus persica	peach	bark	sedative, diuretic
phellandrium	Oenanthe phellandrium	water fennel	fruit	alterative, expectorant
plantago	Plantago ovata	psyllium	seeds	intestinal lubricant

Herb	Latin Name	English Common Name	Plant Part Used	Medicinal Property
polyporus	Polyporus fomentarius	amadou	fungus fruit	arrests local hemorrhages
prunus	Prunus avium	cherry stalks	stalks	astringent tonic
rheum	Rheum palmatum	rhubarb	rhizome	astringent, aperient
scutellaria	Scutellaria laterifolia	skullcap	herb	tonic, nervine
sesamum	Sesamum indicum	sesame	leaves, seeds	demulcent, laxative
sophora	Baptista tinctoria	wild indigo	root, leaves	antiseptic, purgative
uncaria	Uncaria gambier	pale catechu	leaves, shoots	astringent
zanthoxylum	Zanthoxylum americanum	prickly ash	bark, berries	stimulant, tonic
zingiber	Zingiber officinale	ginger	rhizome	stimulant, expectorant
zizyphus	Zizyphus vulgaris	jujube	berries	mucilaginous, pectoral

The following herbs are not well known in Western countries and therefore have no equivalent English names.

akeba
anemarrhena
armeniaca
atractylodes
benincasa
bupleurum
cicoda shell
clutinum
costi
cunidium
dokudami
dulcium
evodia
forsythia
fritillaria
fructus

gastrodia
glehnia
hoelen
moutan
os stegodontis
ostrea testa
pachyma
perilla
phelloptorus
pinella
platycodon
porstythia
rehmannia
schizandra
trichosanthis

APPENDIX C:
Glossary of Medical Terminology

Abdominal. Of the abdomen (belly).

Adenitis. Glandular inflammation.

Adynamia. Lack of vital force as a result of illness.

Alopecia. Baldness.

Aterative. Substance that speeds renewal of tissues after illness.

Amnesia. Partial or total loss of memory caused by brain injury, shock, depression, etc.

Anemia. A condition in which there is a reduction of the number of red blood cells or of the amount of hemoglobin in the blood plasma or both.

Antibilious. Serving to ward off biliousness.

Antiscrofulous. Serving to prevent or cure scrofulosis.

Antiseptic. Serving to prevent infection.

Antispasmodic. Serving to prevent or cure spasms.

Aperient. Serving to produce a natural bowel movement.

Appendicitis. Inflammation of the appendix, a small sac-like outgrowth of the large intestine.

Aromatic. Having an aroma.

Arrhythmia. Any irregularity in the rhythm of the heartbeat.

Arteriosclerosis. A thickening and hardening of the walls of the arteries, as in old age.

Arthritis. Inflammation of a joint.

Asthma. A chronic disorder characterized by wheezing, coughing, difficulty in breathing and a suffocating feeling.

Astringent. Binding. Causing contraction of the tissues.

Atonic Bleeding. Bleeding caused by atony.

Atony. Weakness of the body or of a muscle or organ.

Atrophy. A wasting away of body tissue or an organ, due to insufficient nutrition.

Autointoxication. Poisoning by toxic substances generated within the body.

Basedow's Disease. A disease of the thyroid gland.

Beriberi. A deficiency disease occurring mainly in Asia; caused by a lack of vitamin B_1 in the diet; characterized by extreme weakness, paralysis, anemia, and wasting away.

Bronchitis. An acute or chronic inflammation of the mucous lining of the bronchial tubes. (windpipe).

Caecum. The pouch that is the first part of the large intestine.

Cardiac. Of or near the heart.

Cardiac Asthma. An asthmatic condition dependent on a disease of the heart.

Cardiac Neurosis. A functional disorder of the nervous system that had an effect on the heart.

Carminative. Serving to ease gripping pains and to expel gas from the bowel.

Catarrh. Inflammation of a mucous membrane, especially of the nose or throat, causing an increased flow of mucus.

Cathartic. Serving to produce evacuation of the bowels.

Cerebral. Pertaining to the brain.

Cervical. Of the neck, especially the back of the neck.

Cholecystitis. Inflammation of the gall bladder.

Comedones. Blackheads; plugs of dirt and fatty matter in the skin ducts.

Conjunctivitis. Inflammation of the mucous membrane lining the inner surface of the eyelid.

Constipation. Difficulty in emptying the bowels of waste matter.

Corpulence. Fleshiness of the body.

Coryza. A cold in the head; acute nasal catarrh.

Cystitis. Inflammation of the urinary bladder.

Cystolith. A urinary stony mass.

Debility. Body weakness; feebleness.

Demulcent. Serving to soothe and protect the alimentary canal.

Diabetes. A disease characterized by excessive discharge of urine containing glucose; accompanied by thirst and emaciation.

Diaphoretic. Serving to promote perspiration.

Diarrhea. Excessive frequency and looseness of bowel movements.

Dilatation. Enlargement of an organ cavity or opening of the body beyond its normal size.

Dissipation. Wasteful or excessive indulgence in pleasure and intemperance.

Duodenum. First section of the small intestine between the stomach and the jejunum.

Dyspepsia. Impaired digestion; indigestion.

Eczema. Skin disease with inflammation, itching, and formation of scales.

Edema. Abnormal accumulation of fluid in the tissues or body cavities, resulting in swelling.

Emetic. Serving to cause vomiting.

Emollient. Having a softening and soothing effect.

Empyema. The accumulation of pus in a body cavity, especially the lung cavity.

Endocarditis. Inflammation of the lining of the heart cavities.

Endometritis. Inflammation of the uterus (womb).

Enteritis. Inflammation of the small intestine.

Esophagostenosis. Narrowing of the throat passage.

Ethmoid. Area in the skull through which the olefactory nerves pass.

Expectorant. Serving to promote expectoration and remove secretions from the bronchial tubes.

Febrile. Feverish.

Fermentive Diarrhea. Loose bowel movements, which may be caused by intestinal fermentation as a result of harmful bacteria or deficient gastrointestinal digestive juices.

Frostbite. Injury to a tissue from exposure to intense cold.

Furuncle. A boil.

Gangrene. Decay of body tissue due to obstruction of blood supply.

Gastritis. Inflammation of the stomach, especially the lining.

Gastroenteritis. Inflammation of the lining of the stomach.

Gastroptosis. Downward displacement of the stomach.

Genital. Pertaining to the sex organ.

Graves' Disease. A goiter causing abnormal protrusion of the eyeball; exophthalmic goiter.

Hangover. A condition caused by drinking too much alcoholic beverage.

Heatstroke. A weakened condition caused by exposure to excessive heat.

Hepato-. Having to do with the liver.

Hemiplegia. Paralysis of one side of the body.

Hemoptysis. Spitting up of blood caused by bleeding of the lungs.

Hemorrhage. Heavy bleeding.

Hemorrhoids. Piles.

Hilium. A small opening where vessels or nerves enter an organ.

Hives. See *Urticaria.*

Hydrothorax. Abnormal amount of fluid in the lung cavity.

Hyperacidity. Excess acid in the gastric juice.

Hyperhidrosis. Excessive perspiration.

Hypochondrium. The region on either side of the abdomen just below the lowest rib.

Iliac. Of or near the uppermost of the three sections of the hipbone.

Impotence. Lack of ability to successfully complete sexual intercourse.

Inflammation. A diseased condition of some part of the body, resulting from injury, infection, etc., and characterized by redness, pain, heat, and swelling.

Influenza. An acute contagious infectious disease caused by any of several viruses and characterized by inflammation of the respiratory tract, fever, muscular pain, and often internal disorders; also called grippe, flu.

Insomnia. Inability to sleep.

Inveterate. Long-standing; deep-rooted; firmly established over a long period of time.

Jaundice. A condition in which eyeballs, skin, and urine become abnormally yellow; caused by bile in the blood.

Keratosis. An area of skin marked by overgrowth of horny tissue; a wart.

Lacryoadenitis. Inflammation of the tear ducts.

Laxative. A gentle bowel stimulant.

Leucorrhea. A morbid discharge from the vagina caused by a chronic infection.

Lumbago. Rheumatic pain in the joints; ache in the lower back.

Lymphadenitis. Inflammation of the lymph glands.

Mastitis. Inflammation of the mammary gland (breast).

Menopause. Permanent stopping of menstruation; "change of life."

Migraine. Periodically recurring headache, limited to one side of the head, with nausea, dizziness, etc.

Morning Sickness. Nausea and vomiting occurring in the first months of pregnancy.

Mucus. The thick, slimy secretion of the mucous membrane which serves to moisten and protect those membranes.

Meniere's Disease. A disease or injury probably of the semi-circular canals, characterized by nausea, vomiting, vertigo, deafness, tinnitus aurium, and other phenomena; called also aura and auditory vertigo.

Nausea. Queasiness of the stomach with the impulse to vomit.

Nephritis. Acute or chronic inflammation of the kidney.

Nephrosis. Kidney ailment.

Nephrolithiasis. A condition characterized by the presence of kidney stones.

Nervine. Serving to restore the nerves to their natural state.

Neuralgia. Sudden intense pain extending along the course of a nerve.

Neurasthenia. A neurosis resulting from emotional conflicts; nervous prostration.

Neurogastroenteric. Pertaining to a nerve that serves both the stomach and the intestine.

Neurosis. Any of various psychic or mental disorders.

Nutritive. Nourishing.

Obesity. Excessive body weight due to accumulation of fat in the tissues.

Otitis Media. Inflammation of the middle ear.

Ozena. Foul odor associated with certain cases of atrophic syphilitic ailments and forms of chronic rhinitis. spiration).

Palpitation. Rapid, often irregular, beating of the heart from functional disorder, emotion, etc.

Papillae. Nipplelike protrusions.

Pectoral. Of the chest; relating to or good for diseases of the respiratory tract.

Peristalsis. Rhythmic wavelike motion of the walls of the alimentary canal that moves the contents forward.

Peritonitis. Inflamed lining of the abdominal cavity.

Phlegm. Thick mucus discharge from throat, as during a cold.

Phobia. Irrational fear of a particular object or situation.

Pleurisy. Inflamed lining of the lung area with difficulty in breathing, fever, and dry cough.

Proctocele. Prolapsed rectum, forming a tumor at the anus.

Pruritus. Intense itching of the skin without an eruption.

Pudundal. Pertaining to the external female genitalia.

Purgative. Serving to evacuate the bowels; stronger than a laxative.

Pyrosis. Heartburn.

Rectus Abdominus. Straight muscle of the abdomen.

Refrigerant. Serving to relieve thirst and give a feeling of coolness.

Renal Calculi. Kidney stones.

Rheumatism. Pain in the joints and muscles.

Rhinitis. Inflamed nasal mucous membranes.

Sciatica. Pain along the course of the sciatic nerve in the thighs and legs.

Sclerosis. A hardening of the body tissues or parts, as by an excessive growth of fibrous connective tissue.

Scrofulosis. Tuberculosis of the lymphatic glands of the neck.

Sedative. Serving to calm nervous excitement.

Stricture. Narrowing of a passage in the body.

Stridor. Whistling sound produced in breathing by an obstruction in the bronchial tubes of the lungs.

Smegma. A substance secreted by the sex glands.

Spastic. Muscle spasm.

Sputum. Mucus together with saliva, spat out from the mouth.

Stomachic. Serving to ease disorders of the stomach.

Stomatitis. Inflammation of the mouth.

Sunstroke. Heatstroke caused by excessive exposure to the sun, with high temperature, convulsion, and often coma.

Tachycardia. Abnormally fast heartbeat.
Taenicide. Serving to expel worms.
Tinnitus Aurium. The subjective ringing, whirring, or hissing sound heard in the ears in various afflictions of the eardrum and internal ear; also occurs after taking large doses of certain drugs, notably quinine.
Tonic. Serving to produce a feeling of bodily health.
Tonsillitis. Inflammation of the tonsils.
Tympanitis. Inflammation of the eardrum.

Uremia. A toxic condition of the blood caused by the presence of waste products normally eliminated in the urine; results from an inadequate production of urine.
Urethritis. Inflammation of the urethra.
Urticaria (Hives). An allergic condition characterized by red weltlike swellings of the skin.

Vaginitis. Inflammation of the lining of the vagina.
Vertigo. A sensation of dizziness.
Vesical Calculi. Stones in the urinary bladder.

Wart. A small hard tumor or growth on the skin.
Whooping Cough. Acute infectious disease causing repeated attacks of coughing ending in a "whoop"